Pullingthe**trigger**™

Anxiety, Worry, OCD and Panic Attacks – The Family Edition (Juniors, Teenagers and Parents)
The Definitive **Recovery Approach**

By Adam Shaw and Lauren Callaghan (CPsychol,
PGDipClinPsych, PgCert, MA (hons), LLB (hons), BA)

From the heart and soul of a lifelong OCD and anxiety sufferer, and the expert mind and experience of a leading clinical psychologist, Trigger Press Publishing are proud to introduce the simple yet highly effective self-help method for families (juniors, teenagers and parents and caregivers) – a survival and recovery approach for anxiety, worry, OCD and panic attacks.

The authors

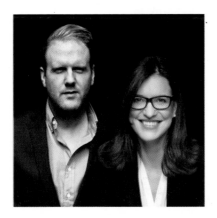

Adam Shaw is a UK philanthropist. Now in recovery from mental health issues himself, he is committed to helping others suffering from debilitating mental health issues through the global charity he co-founded, The Shaw Mind Foundation, www.shawmindfoundation.org.

Lauren Callaghan (CPsychol, PGDipClinPsych, PgCert, MA (hons), LLB (hons), BA), born and educated in New Zealand, is a specialist leading Clinical Psychologist based in London (UK) and the clinic director of two successful private practices which specialise in treating obsessional problems, anxiety disorders, and depression. She is very experienced in working with children, adolescents, and their families across different mental health settings, as well as with adults suffering from anxiety and obsessional problems.

First published in Great Britain 2017 by Trigger Press

Reprinted in 2018 by Trigger Press

Trigger Press is a trading style of Shaw Callaghan Ltd & Shaw Callaghan 23 USA, INC.

The Foundation Centre
Navigation House, 48 Millgate, Newark
Nottinghamshire NG24 4TS UK

www.trigger-press.com

British Library Cataloguing in Publication Data

A CIP catalogue record for this book is available upon request from the British Library

ISBN: 978-1-911246-05-3

This book is also available in the following e-book formats:

MOBI: 978-1-911246-08-4
EPUB: 978-1-911246-06-0
PDF: 978-1-911246-07-7

Cover design, illustrations and typesetting by Fusion Graphic Design Ltd

Printed and bound in Great Britain by Ashford Colour Press, Gosport

Paper from responsible sources

*Dedicated to all the sufferers of any mental health issue and
their loved ones, and to those working tirelessly across all spectrums
around the world to bring a better understanding and awareness of
mental health issues through research, support and treatment.*

> By openly talking about mental health,
> we can pull the trigger on mental illness.

Why have we called our books Pullingthe**trigger**™?

Many things can 'trigger' mental health issues. So what do you do if something makes you feel bad? You stay away from it, right?

I bet you've been avoiding your triggers all your life. But now we know that avoiding your triggers only makes things worse. So here's the game changer: you need to learn how to pull those triggers instead of running away from them – and our **Pulling**the**trigger**™ series shows you how. Your recovery is within reach, we promise.

This is more than recovery, it's a way of life.

Adam Shaw & Lauren Callaghan.

TRIGGERPRESS

Giving mental health a voice

www.trigger-press.com

Thank you for purchasing this book.
You are making an incredible difference.

At least 50% of Trigger Press proceeds go directly to
The Shaw Mind Foundation.

The Shaw Mind Foundation is a charity that focuses entirely on mental health and
was set up by Adam Shaw in order to open conversations around the globe to support sufferers.
It is the parent organisation to Trigger Press, and a large proportion of the proceeds
from the books published go to it. To find out more about The Shaw Mind Foundation
www.shawmindfoundation.org

MISSION STATEMENT

Our goal is to make help and support available for every
single person in society, from all walks of life.
We will never stop offering hope. These are our promises.

Trigger Press and The Shaw Mind Foundation

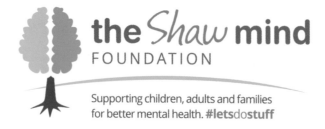

the *Shaw* mind
FOUNDATION

Supporting children, adults and families
for better mental health. #letsdostuff

Contents

Introduction

**Accept Your Mind, Own It For What It Is.
This Takes Courage, Not Fight**

All my life, from being a little boy to a grown man, I tried to suppress my thoughts and anxiety because I knew no better and because I felt compelled to fight them. I was frightened, ashamed, and appalled about my thoughts. My situation was terrifying, lonely, and debilitating. I constantly felt that I was on the edge of madness and no one could help me. It felt like a war I was gradually losing every day as my strength depleted and my energy drained. The day I brought Lauren into my life, some 30 years later, was the day I stopped fighting and my life changed forever. The day I truly accepted my thoughts and embraced them was the day I began to take control. This made surviving my anxiety-based mental illness possible, and more importantly, it made my recovery inevitable. A new life was beginning for me. No words will ever be enough to thank my wife, Alissa, my beautiful children, and of course my therapist and colleague, Lauren Callaghan, for all their unconditional love and support.

Adam Shaw

Adam Shaw: We can all change the game on mental health recovery. It's time for a new way of thinking, so let's make recovery possible for all.

Anxiety and OCD (Obsessive-Compulsive Disorder) have, until quite recently, caused me many difficulties and prevented me from leading a normal life. Although I have helped to raise a large family and been successful in business, my mind has constantly been in turmoil – and all because of the thoughts that have occupied it over the years since I was a small child.

When I was young I worried a lot about all sorts of things – things that might seem silly now. My mind came up with more and more worries and these were very upsetting to me. At first, I worried about bad things happening to my family. Then my worries started telling me that I might be the kind of person who caused bad things to happen to other people. Yet I'm the sort of person who wouldn't harm a fly. I just couldn't understand why I was having 'bad' thoughts. There were many times I thought I was going mad, or that I was a danger to people and had to do certain things so others would be kept safe. For many years, I hid this secret about the workings of my mind. Using a variety of complicated and exhausting techniques, I tried hard to push away my thoughts and get on with being 'normal'. But the harder I pushed, the bigger the problem became. The more I tried to run away and hide, the faster my worries pursued me. It sounds like a horrible nightmare and it was – except I was living this nightmare all day, every day, for a long time.

As you might expect, there is only so long a person can bottle up their worries and anxieties before something dramatic happens. During the period I was fighting anxiety (and, as we will see, 'fighting' is exactly what you shouldn't do!), I had several periods of very poor mental health, the last of which caused me huge distress and led me to think about ending my life. Mentally, I was very troubled indeed, but luckily I sought help from exactly the right person. This was Lauren Callaghan, a highly trained and very experienced therapist who is also co-author of this book.

Why did we decide to write this book?

Having a course of evidence-based therapy finally broke the chains of anxiety that had held me down for so long. However, now I see that if I'd been shown such techniques as a child or a teenager, I would have been able to use them when I was younger, and they would have prevented a lot of distress and difficult periods of anxiety as an adult. This is why I decided, with Lauren, to write a book and share our approach. The techniques I received were so life-changing that I wanted to present them to as many other people suffering from anxiety as possible.

In therapy, Lauren taught me many things that I wished I'd learned when I was much younger and my anxiety was just developing. Perhaps the biggest lesson I learned from her was that I shouldn't fight or run away from my worries. Instead, I should accept them for what they are, embrace them and by doing so, control them. So the three short words which sum up these techniques are:

- **Accept**
- **Embrace**
- **Control**

These three words form the basis of everything Lauren and I will teach you and younger readers in this book. It is a simple, highly effective method and it can work for anyone. It changed my life, and now it can change yours.

- We **accept** that we all have worries and fears, and experience anxiety, and understand that is our current state of mind. We do not question or fight our state of mind; instead, we allow it to be what it is.

- We face our worries and fears, **embrace** them, move towards them and let them in. We do not 'run away' by distracting ourselves, avoiding them or doing other things that we believe will keep ourselves and others 'safe' but which actually cause more problems in the long term.

- We eventually learn how to **control** our mental health and see it for what it is without judging it – a collection of thoughts, feelings and behaviours; no more, no less. 'Control' means accepting that it's okay not to be in control of your thoughts, and the sensations and emotions attached to them.

Our treatment is a combination of Cognitive Behavioural Therapy (CBT) with a Kindness-Focused Approach and it has evolved from the techniques which Lauren introduced me to, as well as our combined experience, wisdom, and expertise. CBT gives us a new way of examining the unhelpful thoughts that we have, helps us look at those thoughts in a different way, and changes our responses. CBT gets easier the more you do it. And we use a very compassionate approach that encourages you to be kind to yourself. Try to remember that we all have unhelpful thoughts, uncomfortable feelings, and strange or problematic behaviours from time to time. So try and be a little less hard on yourself. You have already taken a huge step forward in buying this book, so you can be proud of that.

You'll be pleased to hear that this approach is simple. I'm not a qualified medical person, and the last thing I needed when I was recovering from anxiety and OCD was a lot of confusing information. I needed to be shown a clear path to recovery, and this treatment approach gave me exactly that.

If you follow this approach, even if it might seem uncomfortable at times, you and younger readers will recover. We promise this.

I understand how it feels to be young and worry a lot. I experienced how isolating and lonely it can be. I know what it is like to have troubling thoughts inside your head, and not understand why they're there, or what to do with them. I know what it is like to ask 'Why me?' every day of your life …

I also know that only by accepting and embracing anxiety, worry, and OCD will you ever learn to control them, and stop them ruining your life. Think about it like jumping off a diving board. At first, the fear you have as you stand above the drop feels overwhelming. But you jump, and you realise that it wasn't quite as bad as you thought it was going to be. Then you do it again, and again, and each time you do it, you feel less and less fear. That is how you tackle anxiety, worry, and OCD – by facing it full on. This approach will give you everything you need to rid your mind of the worries, fears, obsessions, and the unhelpful behaviours and compulsions that dominate and ruin your life.

How does this book work?

The book is divided into two parts. In Part I, we will explain to parents, caregivers, and teenagers what anxiety is, and how it can show itself in children and young people. I will share my own story of living with anxiety with you. Then we'll go on to work directly with younger children, using simple language to look at worry and anxiety, and examine the links between thoughts, feelings, and behaviour. We will look at how parents and caregivers can help younger children, and include chapters with a focus on how to tackle OCD in children.

Part II of the book is aimed specifically at children and teenagers, and explains our 'Accept-Embrace-Control' approach in more detail. We have included a section on panic attacks and how to maintain a healthy and positive lifestyle once recovery is underway.

In both sections, we include a range of practical exercises to suit specific age groups, and throughout, we encourage and support parents and caregivers to engage with their child's or teenager's difficulties.

For children, we will use our 'Skeet and Itch' cartoon characters. Skeet is normally a happy, friendly child with good friends and fun hobbies. But quite often, Skeet feels sad. He worries about a lot of things, and suffers with anxiety and OCD. That's where Itch comes in. Itch is all of Skeet's fears and worries, his anxieties, and his OCD represented as a sticky slug that just won't leave Skeet alone. Itch is a heavy burden that won't let Skeet enjoy his life.

Finally, I should just explain why we've called our books about anxiety and OCD *Pulling The Trigger*. You'll be glad to hear that it's nothing to do with guns! Many things 'triggered' my anxiety and OCD but I avoided those triggers, hoping the illness would go away. In fact, avoiding them actually made the illness worse. Now I see that if I'd gone towards those triggers and 'pulled' them – if I'd just faced my fears instead of running away – I would have sorted out my difficulties years ago. Through this book and this approach, I want you to do the same, or encourage younger readers to do it. Good luck everyone on this life-changing journey. Even if it gets tricky, do stay with it. Your recovery is within reach.

We promise.

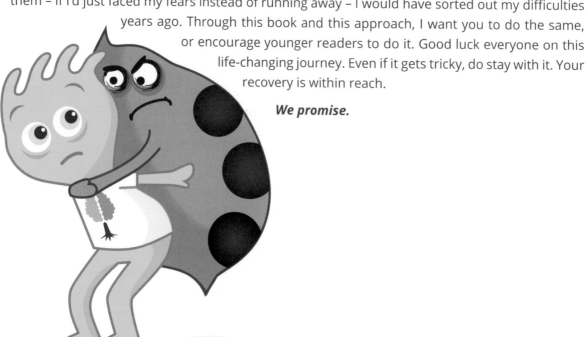

Lauren Callaghan: Hi, I'm Lauren and I'm really pleased that you've picked up this book. It means you've taken a positive step towards your own, or your child's recovery from anxiety, worry, and OCD.

First, a bit about me. I'm originally from New Zealand, where I trained as a clinical psychologist. I was interested in human behaviour and I wanted to be in a profession that helped people, and in which you could see the direct impact of your work in making positive changes for individuals, families, and communities. Eventually, I moved to the UK and I now live in London with my family, where I run two practices specialising in treating a number of disorders, including anxiety and obsessional problems. I have a lot of experience working with children, adolescents, and their families. I have previously worked in secure hospital settings for young people, as well as part of a community and school-based mental health team, working closely with young people, their families, schools, and communities. I went on to specialise in the treatment of anxiety problems, so I understand the difficulties that you and your family are facing, and I'm experienced in developing and promoting age-appropriate treatment for these problems. Our unique treatment approach, which you'll discover in this book, is a very effective approach to the treatment of anxiety, worry, OCD, and panic attacks.

What is WORRY?

In simple terms, worry is when we dwell on things that seem threatening to us in some way. We keep thinking about these things and may go over and over them in our heads. Worry is based on things that haven't actually happened, so we often worry about things that 'might' happen, or things that have already happened, but we can't actually change.

What is anxiety?

Anxiety is a physical and emotional response to worry; to something we consider to be threatening. We all experience anxiety at some point in our lives. When we feel anxious this affects how our body responds, known as the 'fight, flight or freeze' response. 'Fight, flight or freeze' is a very human, very normal way of responding when we feel under threat. In fact, it's been a part of our lives since the time of the cavemen. When they encountered a threat like a terrifying sabre-tooth tiger, they had three choices: they could stand their ground and attempt to fight the tiger, they could run away as fast as their hairy legs could carry them, or they could freeze and hope the tiger would pass them by in favour of tastier prey. That's fight, flight or freeze in a nutshell.

The words 'anxiety', 'fear' and 'worry' are often used interchangeably, but here's what we mean when we talk about anxiety, fear and worry in this book:

- Worries are the thoughts you have about a future event, real or imagined, that scare you. Or they can be about things that have happened that we can't change.
- Fear is the emotional reaction to real or perceived imminent danger.
- Anxiety describes the emotions (including fear and physiological sensations) that we have in response to what we anticipate as a threat.

What is OCD?

My definition of OCD is that it's an obsessional problem that can be about anything, causing us to feel anxious, depressed, ashamed, and guilty. In brief, OCD is when people have uncontrollable, upsetting thoughts called intrusions which they interpret as threatening. This makes them feel worried, anxious, and fearful. Naturally, they want to minimise or reduce the threat by doing something. This may be a compulsion or ritual, or some other 'safety behaviour'.

What are intrusions?

Intrusions are thoughts, or images or doubts, or even feelings, urges or sensations that are uncontrollable. Not all intrusions are unwanted, e.g. having an image pop into your head about your last holiday on the beach. But in OCD, intrusive thoughts are unwanted and very unpleasant. For example, you might have an image pop into your head of someone close to you dying, or have an intrusive feeling that things are just 'not right' which suddenly overwhelms you.

What are obsessions?

Obsessions are the upsetting intrusions in OCD, which as we've said, can be thoughts, or images or doubts, or even feelings, urges or sensations. These might include thoughts of harming yourself or others, having the urge to push someone down the stairs, having doubts that you did a certain thing properly, having thoughts that something bad will happen because of something you did or didn't do, or worries about things being out of order. (Of course, this is only a tiny list; the number of things people can fixate on is practically infinite.)

What are compulsions?

Compulsions, also known as rituals, are the things we do (or don't do) to reduce or eliminate intrusions or stop the feared outcome from happening. These might include excessive handwashing or cleaning, checking and tidying, repeating words silently, avoiding people or certain situations, collecting items, or seeking reassurance from other ritualised actions such as turning switches on and off. (Remember, this not an exhaustive list.) We do these things because we believe in some way that they keep things stable and safe.

What are safety behaviours?

Safety behaviours are the behaviours we rely on when we have an anxiety problem because we believe that they will protect us from the feared consequence. They often include avoidance (when people try to avoid the thoughts, feelings and situations that frighten them in the hope it will keep them 'safe') or seeking reassurance from people to confirm or reject a supposition or belief. In OCD, safety behaviours include compulsions and rituals.

What are panic attacks?

Panic attacks are short-lived but very intense experiences of anxiety building up in our bodies. They can be terrifying and overwhelming, and people experience the physical signs of fear and anxiety, including increased heart rate, shallow breathing, feeling hot and sweaty, dizziness, and feeling sick. They can happen out of the blue for no apparent reason, or as part of a worrying situation. During a panic attack, people often worry that something is wrong with them and / or that a panic attack will happen again suddenly, so do their best to stop this from happening.

Why do we experience anxiety?

Anxiety is a perfectly natural response to a threatening situation and we all experience it from time to time. It is a fundamental part of being human, and we cannot banish it permanently just because at some points in our lives it misfires and becomes a problem. What we can do instead is manage it so that it doesn't become a bigger problem than it needs to be.

We understand that, as a parent, it is very difficult to watch your child suffering from anxiety. The need to respond in a way which removes the anxiety completely is overwhelming. But please remember: **anxiety is normal**. It is nature's way of responding to a threat, and it prompts the 'fight, flight or freeze' mechanism (explained in more detail in Chapter 5) which is very useful indeed in difficult situations.

So if you are experiencing anxiety, or you're the parent of a child who is, you are by no means alone. There are millions of people in the same boat, all trying to figure out why they feel bad and what they can do to stop the feeling. For most of us, anxiety is only a fleeting problem – a response to giving a talk in class, or an annual trip to the dentist, for example. For others, it is a severe issue; a persistent, chronic problem that negatively affects many parts of their lives.

It is normal, as a parent, to not only feel sympathy for your child as they struggle with anxiety, but also to feel guilty for the part you think you may have played in causing it. However, please try not to blame yourself. It is not helpful for you or them, and it won't help your child overcome it. Anxiety problems develop for many reasons and they are common.

Estimates suggest that up to 10 per cent of all children have an anxiety problem. As a parent, you may have anxiety too, which might make it difficult for you to engage with our treatment plan because you want to protect and reassure your child about the things they find distressing (which might be things you find distressing too!) Again, this is perfectly normal. If you are in this situation it may be worth looking at our companion book for adults (**Pulling the Trigger**: The definitive survival and recovery approach for OCD, anxiety, panic attacks and related depression) to help you understand how to manage anxiety for yourself.

Our treatment method uses 'exposure' techniques which allow the child or young person to experiment with and confront their fears, and see them for what they are: essentially, just thoughts that are scary, or worrying thoughts about events that haven't happened, or are unlikely to happen, or are unlikely to be as awful as they imagine. However, this does not mean we will force children into situations that they do find scary – that might make the problem even worse! Instead, we work in a graduated way, teaching children with anxiety that only by facing fear do we ever conquer it.

For example, a child who is frightened of dogs would understandably have a meltdown if they were put in a room with a barking Alsatian or Rottweiler. But they might start to understand that not all dogs are threatening if they're encouraged to give a friendly poodle a pat on the head.

On the subject of dogs, perhaps we should mention that family behaviour around a child with anxiety problems can actually make the anxiety worse. If, say, your child is scared of dogs, you may seek to alleviate their worry by not going anywhere as a family that will involve encounters with dogs. By reassuring the child that you won't encounter a dog, it doesn't just reinforce the fear that all dogs are dangerous and out to attack, but it severely restricts what the family can do socially. In a nutshell, it becomes the whole family's problem – and it can apply to many different forms of anxiety. So in this book we encourage parents and caregivers to think about how their child's anxiety is affecting patterns of family life, how they might be facilitating this, and how to manage it for the benefit of everyone.

FOR TEENAGERS

Over 13? Then I think you might prefer to work through this book yourself. It's worth it. It'll give you a whole new understanding about your anxiety problem as a result. You might need a little extra help from a therapist, or someone you trust who'll listen to you without making judgements. This might be a parent or caregiver, but it could be a teacher, a school counsellor, or a relative. The first thing we ask you to do is read Adam's story in the next chapter. See if some or all of his story sounds familiar to you. Hopefully it will. After that, you'll move on to your own dedicated section in Part II. We completely understand that dealing with anxiety, worry, and OCD is scary and difficult. As a teenager, you already have a lot going on in your life, and the last thing you need is a big extra dose of worry and fear. You're probably feeling alone and isolated, and you think that no one understands how you feel, or why you're worried. You're trying to pretend that you're okay, that things are normal and that no one will notice how bad you're feeling. And that can be exhausting. It's scary and it's difficult, and it is messing around with your life. But there is help out there. This book can help you manage your anxieties and see them for what they are: a collection of thoughts, feelings, and bodily sensations. While they might seem unpleasant, that is all they are.

Finally, parents and caregivers need to spend time reading this book, understanding what anxiety is and how it applies to their child, then working though each section carefully. That can be a big ask when you have busy working lives and possibly other children to see to. But if you can devote just a bit of time every day, you'll soon see the benefits. Our approach is not complicated but it does require dedication and commitment. As a parent, you will need to be your child's guide.

The next chapter is Adam's story. He tells us about the difficulties he experienced with anxiety, worry, and OCD from childhood up to his late teens. This chapter is an essential read. Adam's personal experience inspired this book and he knows, first-hand, exactly what it is like to suffer from extreme anxiety as a child and teenager.

I can't promise it will always be easy. If it was then you probably wouldn't need to read this book at all. It is challenging and it requires patience, perseverance, and trust. However, if you approach this book and treatment method with an open mind you will see results and you WILL get better, just as Adam did, just at the point when he thought all hope had been lost.

Good luck on your journey, and stay with it!

Part I

Adam Shaw – My Story

Chapter 1

My Battle with Worry

My name is Adam Shaw, and I was born in the UK city of Sheffield in 1977. Our family is an ordinary one – my dad was a builder and my mum worked in a bank. My dad came from one of the poorest parts of Sheffield but worked hard to build a business. Compared to other people in the area we were comfortably off. When I was younger I enjoyed holidays abroad, nice clothes, and brand new trainers. Saying that, my mum and dad made me understand the value of money, and how hard work brings rewards in life.

I was a secure and happy child with no obvious difficulties and I certainly didn't feel 'different' to other people. I didn't have any issues with either of my parents and I can't find any reason to think we were anything other than a normal family.

If I'm asked about my earliest memories I can remember opening my first ever Spider-Man toy on Christmas Day, or proudly wearing my new football kit. But my strongest memories, which began to form around the age of five, are of my developing anxiety.

Little worries

I started school at the age of five. Like most children that age, I was accompanied on the journey to school by my parents. In my case, this was almost always my mum. For some reason, I developed the idea that my mum would be in danger after she'd dropped me off, and that she might be harmed on her way home.

This left me feeling sad, anxious and worried.

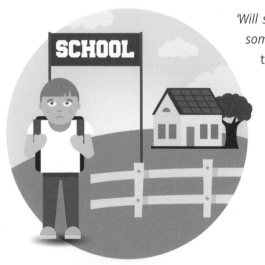

'Will she pick me up from school?' I wondered, 'or will she be dead somewhere? What will I do then?' I fretted over what might happen to her when she was out of my sight.

I couldn't figure out what might happen if she didn't pick me up. I was doing well at school and making friends. Outwardly everything was okay, but inside I felt sad – really sad and worried – and I couldn't understand why that was.

I noticed that my worries were beginning as soon as I woke up in the morning. An uneasy feeling would creep over me the minute I opened my eyes. It made me want to cry.

'What will happen today?'

'Will Mum be killed or injured?'

'This feels horrible. How can I stop feeling so bad?'

These thoughts nagged me and I couldn't shake them off. Then, by chance, I discovered a little routine that suddenly made everything feel okay again. I noticed that if I looked under my bed four times before getting out of it – twice on one side, twice on the other – everything that day would be just fine. There were four members of our family: mum, dad, myself, and sister Lauren, so doing things four times made sense.

And it was always four. If I counted wrong, I'd have to start again. But if I got it right, I would feel bright and happy and I'd have no worries. This lasted for a while and I was pleased I'd found something that made me feel better. I did not know, but this was the beginning of my Obsessive Compulsive Disorder (OCD).

'Look at the clouds!'

Later, we will learn that anxiety, worry, and OCD have a nasty way of getting past rituals designed to make you feel better, by turning them into ones which no longer work. So one day, just after I'd arrived at school, I became anxious and worried about my mum as she left to go home. Although I'd done the 'four times' ritual, for some reason it hadn't worked that day.

Then I caught a glimpse of a cloud, high above the school. And this is what I thought:

'I've just seen a big cloud. No one else has seen it but me, and if no one else sees it something bad will happen to my mum.'

I don't know why I chose clouds. It doesn't really matter. What counts is that I'd attached an **importance** to them, a meaning that spelled disaster. I knew that in seconds, the cloud would change shape and never look the same again. I needed someone else to look at it, and quickly.

I turned to my school mates. 'Look at the clouds!' I shouted, 'look at the clouds!' Puzzled, they looked up. 'They're just clouds,' one of them said. 'So what?'

I didn't explain, but immediately I felt better because they'd seen it too. And for about two years I did the same thing, every single day. I must have driven my friends mad, but they always did what I asked, and they even turned it into a joke.

My worries and anxieties began to interfere with my life, particularly sport. Some of the hardest times I had with the 'clouds' worry was during PE in the school playground. I dreaded going out to play football on a dull day in case I caught sight of the clouds.

The other boys would be too involved in the game to take any notice of me asking them to look up at the sky, and if my teacher caught me turning one of my friends' heads upwards (which I sometimes did) I got into trouble. This became agony for me, particularly if I needed to 'head' the ball towards the goal. My dad would come to watch me playing for the school team and he noticed my reluctance to head the ball.

'What's the matter, son?' he asked. 'Are you scared of it hurting you?'

I nodded in agreement. But I wasn't scared of the ball at all; I was scared of seeing the clouds, and the message of doom that they seemed to carry.

The clouds worry must have lasted two years or more, and all that time I was tormented by thoughts that bad things would happen to my family. As parents or caregivers we're sometimes too quick to dismiss such thoughts as silly nonsense but as children – particularly those who are sensitive to the world around them – worries and anxieties can be hard to shake off.

There were times when I saw clouds and others didn't, yet nothing bad happened to my mum or anyone else in my family. Now I know that there is no connection between seeing clouds (or anything else) and bad things happening to loved ones, but I just didn't make that connection then. I was stuck in a loop of worry and fear.

Even at home, and with my mum around, the clouds obsession still nagged me. The summer holidays were a nightmare. With my classmates scattered for the full six weeks, there were few other kids around who could see the clouds with me. For days and weeks I'd keep my head low, making sure I didn't look up at the sky.

It was very hard to keep this up for such a long time, and I became so low, miserable and worried that eventually I decided to tell my mum. As you might expect, my explanation about clouds and bad things happening sounded, to adult ears, just plain silly. Remember that this was in the days when anxiety, worry, and OCD didn't have the awareness it does today.

'Now Adam,' my mum said, 'you really mustn't start thinking like that and wishing bad things on yourself. That's how people end up in mental hospitals.'

She meant well. Generally, most parents and caregivers mean well, even if what they say doesn't always come out the right way. I don't blame my mum at all for saying it. She was only trying to help.

And it worked – but for all the wrong reasons. I started to worry about mental hospitals. I'd heard about these places – big, scary old buildings full of padded cells and mad people wandering about in their nightclothes, screaming and crying. In fact, there was one such place near us that was feared locally as somewhere you might end up in if you were a 'lunatic'.

So far from making me feel better, the idea that I might end up in a madhouse caused even more anxiety. Just thinking about it made me feel sick with worry.

'Oh my God,' I thought, 'I can't end up there. I'll really not have to look at the clouds now.'

From day to day I was trying to live a normal life, but most of the time I just felt as though a deep, dark gloom was hanging over me. It was a daily battle to remain cheerful and unworried.

Chapter 2

It's All My Fault!

As I grew a bit older, the clouds obsession faded, but I still believed something bad would happen if I didn't carry out my 'four times' ritual regularly. I had to switch lights on and off four times, taps on and off four times. And if I got anything 'wrong', e.g. only turning the light off three times instead of four, I'd have to do the whole thing over again. Before and after every football match I played in, I'd have to do four 'kick-ups' with the ball each time. This ritual became worse during the times I was on my own, and even when it wasn't there, I always had a 'heavy' feeling that it would soon come back. Just having a bath became a ritual, in that I had to turn on the hot tap in four-second bursts. It was dominating my life and causing a lot of distress.

I must stress that, on the surface, I was a normal kid. This makes it quite difficult for parents to spot the signs of anxiety, worry, and OCD. I was just like anyone else my age; I had a sense of humour, I loved sport, I liked hanging out with my friends. I was normal. Yet inside I felt a mess, and no matter how hard I tried, this mess was always around to haunt me.

'All my fault'

One summer, when I was around 10 or 11, I went on a camping trip with my best friend, Chris, and his parents. On the Sunday, just a few hours before we were due to go home, we headed for the woods close by the camp. We'd taken a box of matches from a tent and, as boys do, we were playing with them, striking them before quickly blowing them out.

'We'd better leave some in the box,' Chris said, 'so my mum and dad won't suspect we've been playing with them.'

As we reached the edge of the wood, on the way back to the camp, Chris inspected the box.

'I'm sure there were more left in here than this,' he said. 'Maybe some have dropped out?'

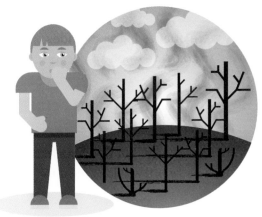

'Maybe,' I said. Then, a huge wave of panic and fear swept over me like I'd never experienced before.

'We've left live matches in the woods,' I thought. *'What happens if they catch fire, the trees burn down and all the animals are killed?'*

I felt sick with fright and anxiety. 'Come on,' I said to Chris, 'we'll have to go back and pick them all up!'

We retraced our steps but found no unused matches. That might have told me that we hadn't actually dropped any. Instead, it only fuelled my anxiety, causing me to think that somehow we'd missed them.

On the drive home, I was completely silent. All I could think about were the trees going up in flames and animals burning to death. And I would be responsible for that.

Panic attacks

When I arrived home I told my mum I wasn't feeling well, and went to bed. But I couldn't sleep. I felt sick with fear. I lay awake, shaking and sweating. I had no idea what was wrong with me. After a few minutes I calmed down, but then the thing returned, doubled in strength. I felt I was going crazy – just as my mum had predicted. In fact, in the months ahead I would refer to it as my 'crazy situation'. Of course, looking back, I know that I was experiencing my first panic attack.

Sleepless nights

The feelings I had were horrible, and often they were accompanied by sleepless nights. I lay there wondering what was happening to me, and why. My worries were really interfering with my sleep and the more I worried, the more my sleep patterns went haywire. I would wake up in the night, and immediately the scary thoughts would leap in. I didn't wake up feeling relaxed in the morning; a bad night's sleep only made matters worse.

These sickening feelings and the disturbed sleep went on for a few days. Finally, I plucked up the courage to watch the news and scan through the evening newspapers. There wasn't a single mention of a fire anywhere in the area I'd been camping. I breathed a sigh of relief. I was off the hook. I wondered why I'd been so concerned about it in the first place.

The not-so-lucky kid

My world settled down again – until we went on holiday to Florida later that year. Going abroad with my family, plus my auntie, uncle and cousins, was a really big treat. I was a huge basketball fan and loved everything about America, from sports to training shoes to music. I was hugely excited about going and couldn't wait to get there.

We went to Disneyland and the theme park was packed. There were queues for all the rides. In one queue, I saw a disabled boy in a wheelchair who was allowed to go to the front, and get on the ride before everyone else.

'Lucky kid,' I thought jealously.

As soon as I had this thought, it came into my head that I was terrible for thinking like that. That boy had a physical disability. It wasn't his fault. And he was far from being 'lucky'. But the thought wouldn't go away. From then on, every time I saw a disabled person, a bad word would come into my head; a word like 'bastard'. A terrible word to describe anyone.

After the rides, we went for a meal at a nearby restaurant. I felt destroyed by my thoughts, couldn't eat and said I wasn't feeling very well.

'Straighten your face,' said my dad. 'We've come all this way for a nice holiday and I don't want to see you sulking.'

'Sorry, Dad,' I said, not wanting to share the real reason for my moodiness.

I desperately wanted to be happy, but my head was buzzing with terrible thoughts. Then I saw a group of old people going by.

'They're bastards, too,' I thought. *'I hope they die.'*

Now I was really tormented by my thoughts, and there was no escape. Wherever I saw people with disabilities and elderly people, my thoughts got worse, the more I tried to push them away. I tried repeating the phrase 'don't think, don't think, don't think' again and again, even muttering it to myself so that I wouldn't be heard.

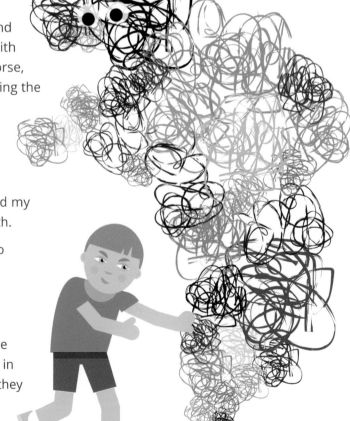

But I was heard.

'Hey Adam, what's that you're mumbling?' asked my uncle. He'd spotted me muttering under my breath.

'Oh, it's nothing,' I replied. 'I'm just pretending to be a robot ...'

In short, I was going to great pains to disguise my fears.

Did my thoughts about the elderly and people with disabilities go away once my family's holiday in America was over? No, they didn't. If anything, they got worse.

Chapter 3

Don't Wish Bad Things ...

At the age of 11, I moved from primary school to senior school; a huge jump in terms of the number of pupils and the level of work involved. I was taking a leap from a cosy bubble into something unknown and potentially scary.

It was a very big school, and very diverse in terms of its pupils' backgrounds. It was the first time I'd come up against kids who had all kinds of challenges in life. It was the first time I'd seen a real fist-fight between boys, and the level of violence shocked me. How would I cope?

The answer is: actually quite well. Although I was the youngest in my year, I had a quality about me that helped me to fit in. As I've mentioned, I was good at sports and I wasn't shy or nervous. I'd go out of my way to avoid trouble, but I knew I could look after myself if necessary.

All the stuff on the surface was fine. But inside my head, everything was haywire. I discovered that I was always watching out in case I saw elderly people or people with disabilities and had a bad thought about them. The worry that I might have a thought like, 'I hope you die, you old bastard' tormented me. I was so scared of that sentence that I would do anything to get it out of my head.

'Don't wish bad things ...'

The only answer, I thought, was to avoid the elderly and people with disabilities altogether. I'd always enjoyed seeing my grandparents; now I tried to make excuses for not visiting them, or not being in when they came around. During this period a couple of kids from school lost their dads in tragic circumstances. I was friends with them both, but I avoided them in case something bad came out of my mouth. They must have thought I was awful, but I was more worried about what I'd say to them.

Soon, I developed a little phrase to help me through these periods, which was 'Adam, don't wish bad things upon yourself'. As you'll remember, that was adapted from what my mum had said to me. She'd added the words '...or you'll end up in a mental hospital' but I tried not to think about that part. So if I said, 'don't wish bad things' to myself, I was able to deal with the thought and block it out at the same time. Perfect. Or so I thought.

You know that feeling when you do something so many times that it doesn't mean much anymore? Well, that's what happened to me after repeating 'don't wish bad things upon yourself' countless times. At the start, it made me feel comfortable for a few days. Then that went down to a day, then hours, then minutes. I had to keep saying it over and over again until I felt better.

And I was still doing the 'four times' ritual constantly, hoping that its 'magic' would also help to keep the bad things from happening, and keep the nasty thoughts at bay. All this stuff going on in my head was tiring and eventually it began to affect my schoolwork. I found it hard to concentrate, not because I was lazy or didn't understand, but because my mind was occupied by the rituals keeping the bad thoughts away.

To everyone else, it looked like I WAS lazy and didn't understand. I heard my mum telling someone that my sister was 'the academic one', not me. She didn't mean it nastily at all, but there was a reason for my failure in school, something I couldn't discuss with anyone. Every minute in the classroom was hell. There was always a battle going on in my head between my horrible thoughts and getting through the lesson.

All the time I was desperately trying to figure out what was happening to me. And asking myself:

'Should I tell my parents?'
'Should I see a doctor?'
'Where do I find help?'

I didn't tell my parents. I thought they wouldn't understand. And I daren't go to the doctor in case I was diagnosed as 'mad' and sent to a mental hospital. For me, it seemed the only option was to sort it out myself. Every time I saw my school friends I'd wish I was them. 'Look at them,' I'd think, 'they've no worries at all. I wish I could be normal.' All I wanted to do was go to the park, play football and never have a bad thought about another person ever again. It didn't seem too much to ask.

'Could I be the same?'

In 1993, when I was in my mid-teens, something dreadful happened that shifted my anxiety, worry, and OCD up several gears. In Liverpool, a toddler called James Bulger was abducted by two 10-year-old boys, who murdered him on a railway line. The whole country was shocked and appalled, and for weeks this terrible incident was all over the TV news and in the papers.

Where I lived there were many little kids the same age as James Bulger. By then, I was tall and well built. Physically, I could easily kill a two year old, if I'd wanted to. And that's where my new difficulties began: the thought of being capable of killing a toddler preyed on my mind so much that I began to think I had the potential to be a murderer.

Imagine how that must have felt ...

Day after day, night after night, I had terrible thoughts about killing children. I had no access to weapons, but neither had the boys who killed James Bulger. They had done it with their bare hands, and so could I. The horror of knowing this preyed on my mind:

Could I do it?
Would I do it?
Who would be my victims?
Could I strangle my sister, or my mum?

These thoughts went round and round, like some terrible ghost train fairground ride.

Later that year the neighbourhood I lived in was rocked by the killing of a postman on his round. He was run over by robbers who stole his mail, and he was the first ever postman to be killed in the UK while on duty.

This was just before Christmas, and unsurprisingly it was a huge event in our area. The police and TV cameras were everywhere – nothing like this had ever happened round our way before. It was shocking – and, of course, it preyed on my mind.

I thought about it so much that I started to wonder whether I'd actually carried out the attack. That sounds crazy, doesn't it? If anyone had been listening to my thoughts, they'd have laughed out loud but I really started to convince myself that I could've done it. I even thought I might have somehow been sleepwalking. The worry started to grind me down. I felt like a hollow-eyed wreck.

I believed I was a terrible risk to other people, as well as to myself. I tried to think of ways to stop myself from attacking people. Later on, I even bought a pair of handcuffs that I would keep in my pocket in case I had an urge to strangle someone, and I could lock myself up before I acted on the urge. I tried to calm myself with the 'don't wish bad thoughts' mental ritual, but I kept having to say it over and over again until the thought went away.

And it didn't take long before it came back. When it happened I could feel a tingling in my hands and I convinced myself it was a sure sign that I was a potential murderer. Even something as simple as a pen lying on a desk sent me into a worry that I could pick it up and stab the boy sitting next to me. In fact, I became so nervous around pens that I somehow convinced my classmates to help me with my written work.

Struggling to make sense of it all

It won't surprise you to learn that I left school with very few qualifications. However, I got on to a sports course at a local college, met new people, and started to enjoy life a bit more. I used to go out on Tuesday nights with a group of friends and I'd find that drinking alcohol took my mind off my worries. But when you're young, one drink can sometimes lead to more and I'd find that hangovers made my anxieties much worse.

The silly thing is that, deep down, I knew I wasn't a murderer or a psychopath. But my thoughts were telling me otherwise, and I just couldn't understand that. Why would I want to ruin my life by wishing to kill someone, when I wasn't even a violent person? I couldn't figure that out at all, and it took me many years before the penny dropped that what I was worrying about was the thought itself – nothing more. It was only then that I realised that, by trying to stop the bad things from happening, and by trying so hard to understand why I was having all these upsetting thoughts, I was actually making it worse.

All the time I was having bad thoughts, I was in turmoil. Outwardly I might have been positive, happy-go-lucky, and fun, but inside, it was a different story. I thought my 'bad thoughts' would last forever, and nothing would or could take them away. And when you're young, that's a terrible burden to carry around.

Chapter 4

Back from the Brink

During my time at college I met a girl who eventually became my girlfriend. Our relationship didn't last too long, but during the time I was with her, I noticed that my anxiety and OCD wasn't nearly as bad as it had been. There were moments when I felt it had returned, but on the whole, it seemed to fade into the background.

You can find a much fuller account of my difficulties with anxiety, worry, and OCD beyond my teenage years in the adults' version of this book. So let me just say that I was poorly for a long time. But then I met the girl who eventually became my wife, and we started a family. I worked for a firm of solicitors, before leaving to start my own business. I worked very hard to establish myself, and in time became very successful.

All the time I was working and helping to look after my family, my anxieties took control. There were periods when the anxiety lessened, but generally, every day was a battle to manage the bad thoughts I was having.

Back from the brink

Eventually, I became very unwell as a result of anxiety, worry, and OCD. It had got me again. I was desperate. I felt as if I had no one to turn to. And that's when I decided to kill myself.

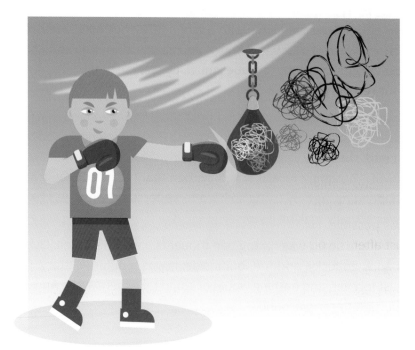

I almost went through with it. I got as far as the bridge, but something – a little bit of hope, perhaps – pulled me back from the brink.

Not long afterwards, I met Lauren and eventually, with her help, I got better. I know I'm not – and never will be – 100 per cent free from anxiety, worry, and OCD.

But accepting that is the first step towards recovery. I'm certainly in a much better place than I was before I met Lauren, now that I have learned to accept and embrace my worries.

In this book, you will learn – as I did – to **accept** and **embrace** your anxiety, your worry, and your OCD. You will NOT be encouraged to 'battle with' or 'fight' your difficulties, because that does not work. I battled and fought constantly, and got nowhere.

The moment you accept and embrace worries and unpleasant or scary thoughts and uncomfortable feelings, you change the game. And the new rules of the game are that **you are in control, not your illness**. Lauren taught me to face my fears and worries, and accept them. If I did, she said, those fears and worries would become less important and I would get better.

When you face your fears head-on, you will feel better. I promise this. You take control by not having control. What I mean by that is when you recognise you have a problem with anxiety, worry, and OCD, instinctively you want to find out what it is, what has caused it and how you can go about fixing it.

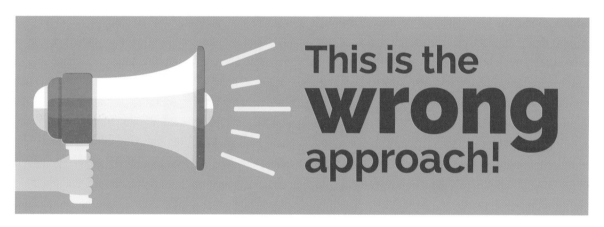

THIS IS THE WRONG APPROACH!

I cannot state this loudly enough! Stop asking 'why' and just accept what is. No matter how you feel, accept it. It won't cure you, but in my opinion this is the fundamental foundation for beginning your recovery.

During our therapy sessions together I saw how 'accepting' was empowering, not the other way round. And the more I sat with anxiety, worry, and OCD, and even welcomed them in like old friends, the more I faced them down. They had no power over me any more.

Knowing this was like discovering a miracle. It was my 'lightbulb moment'; finding out about it led me through the dark path and out into a world where recovery from anxiety, worry, and OCD was possible. I was so pleased to feel this way that I started to fulfil a promise I made to myself just after the time I got so close to committing suicide.

'Adam,' I said, *'if you ever recover from this, or find a way through it, you will do something about it and pass it on. You will not recover in silence. You will be public about it, and by exposing it, you will help other people suffering in the same way. You will make your wife and children proud.'*

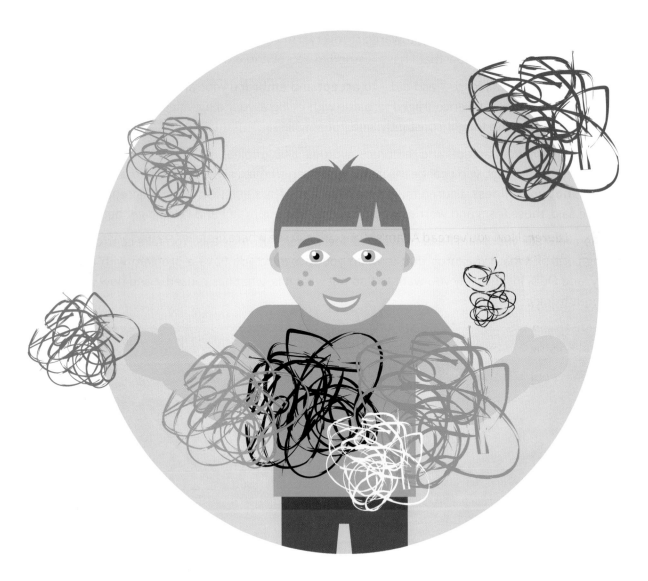

And so this is where I am today; publishing books on mental health and overcoming adversity. Working with my own charity and helping people like you to understand that what you're going through is not unusual, and that you are not weird, freaky, odd or anything else just because you're suffering from anxiety, worry, and OCD.

We can make our mental health issues the biggest positive influence in our life. If approached correctly, our mental health problems can actually give us the platform we need to take action and create a fulfilling life for the future. In reality, our mental health issues have created and given us a strength we did not know we had; a sense of resilience. Think about it – you already have a 100 per cent success rate even before beginning this recovery approach. You have survived every day no matter how bad the distress or torment has been.

Use this view of your strength to drive your courage forward in embracing our new recovery approach. Accept and embrace your mental health issues and thank them for allowing you to learn from them. Life is there for the taking; go to it and embrace every moment of it.

Chapter 5

The Anxiety Behind the Worries

 Lauren: Now you've read Adam's story, and can see where his fears started and how they developed, let's look a little more closely at the anxiety which lay beneath his worries and OCD.

As I mentioned in the Introduction, anxiety, far from being a problem, is actually a **normal human reaction** to something we perceive as a threat. For example, if we're out walking and we see a big dog running towards us barking, we're likely to react in two ways:

• The first is our emotional reaction, which might be one of immediate fear, or even panic.

• The second is our physical reaction. We might start to sweat and shake, and feel our stomach turning over.

No matter that the dog might just run past and pay us no attention; we have responded instinctively to what we perceive as a threat. This is our 'fight, flight or freeze' response kicking in. So what do we do next?

1) Do we stand our ground (**'fight'**) and hope the dog backs off?

2) Do we run away (**'flight'**) before it reaches us?

3) Or do we just stay there (**'freeze'**) hoping it runs past and doesn't notice us?

What is fight, flight or freeze?

This is a response that has its roots in prehistoric times, when early man faced dangerous predators that would kill him for food if they got the chance. Despite being an animalistic survival response, 'fight, flight or freeze' has stayed with us right up to the present day. When we're faced with some kind of a threat, we get the same surge of adrenaline – that's what makes us feel brave and gives us the extra strength to fight, or the extra speed to run away, while the freeze response allows us to hear and see everything with greater clarity. So fight, flight or freeze is a wonderful tool – a protective response to help keep us safe.

There's just one problem. Fight, flight or freeze makes more sense when the threat is obvious. A big dog running towards us has the potential for threat. An even bigger threat was the prehistoric sabre-toothed tiger prowling around outside a cave – so the cavemen inside either hid or agreed to join together and fight it off.

There are a number of physical sensations you may experience associated with the physiological changes in the body due to the fight, flight or freeze response.

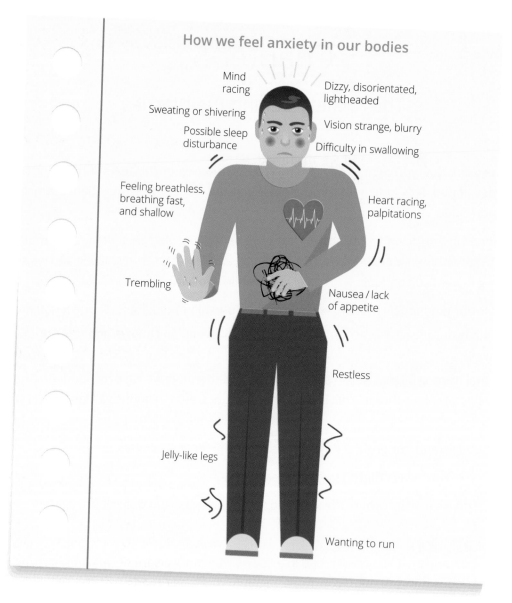

How we feel anxiety in our bodies

Mind racing

Dizzy, disorientated, lightheaded

Sweating or shivering

Vision strange, blurry

Possible sleep disturbance

Difficulty in swallowing

Feeling breathless, breathing fast, and shallow

Heart racing, palpitations

Trembling

Nausea / lack of appetite

Restless

Jelly-like legs

Wanting to run

Today, threats aren't always so obvious. As well as being physical, such as the dog or sabre-toothed tiger, they can be mental and emotional too. And though we respond to the threat in the way we always did, with 'fight, flight or freeze', it can be harder now to say exactly what that threat is.

Threats faced today

For example, giving a presentation in class or encountering a negative comment about ourselves on Facebook or Twitter could cause as much anxiety, relatively speaking, as the sabre-toothed tiger did to our cavemen ancestors. This threat won't kill you, but it is a threat in today's world, because being rejected or made fun of is a challenge to our social standing and might cause us to become shy or withdraw from friends. It might lead us to under-perform at school, and worry about what people think of us. These responses are perfectly normal because **anxiety is normal and everyone experiences it** – even those who always seem to be so calm on the outside experience anxiety.

That said, anxiety becomes a problem if we are experiencing it too frequently and / or too intensely in specific situations and we don't manage it as well as we should. Anxiety creates worries we experience regularly, to the point we feel they are part of our everyday lives. If a barking dog running towards us has caused us anxiety, we might start to worry about what will happen next time we encounter that dog. And we might extend this to worry about what will happen the next time we see any dog. So the worry has grown from a simple response to a barking dog into one that takes in all dogs, barking or not. Adam had an anxious moment when he combined a bad thought about his mum with the appearance of a cloud. Then his worries grew into ones about his mother being hurt or killed. At the root of these worries is the idea that 'something bad' will happen. You might not always know exactly what that bad thing is, but you can have an overwhelming feeling of dread that something bad will happen, or is about to happen.

All children experience anxiety – it's a perfectly normal part of a child's development that helps them develop the skills they need to deal with situations that scare them. So worries are a common part of a child's life. For pre-teen children, common worries include their performance at school, their relationships with friends, their health, and fears about dying and losing people close to them.

The focus of their worries will change as children get older. Without even knowing it, younger children experience very immediate threats relating to their own survival; so they may experience a fear of loud noises or strangers. As they get older, their fear may progress to a fear of losing their caregivers; later, it may centre on a fear of rejection from their friends. Rejection can mean loss of social status or being part of a group – something that has been part of our survival instinct as a species.

Worries like these are all very normal, and worries will be personal to each person's experiences. A child who grows up on a busy main road in a city may be more aware of cars and crossing roads than his / her cousin in the country who is frightened of busy roads. Yet the city child might have unspecified worries about fields and farm animals that his cousin doesn't think twice about. Equally, there could be a touch of anxiety in each child's responses to their own environments which keeps them aware and safe.

So there are positive benefits to anxiety and it's worth saying again that **anxiety is completely normal**. It only starts to become a problem when it interferes in our lives in some significant way. For young people, this can affect attendance at school or training courses, study, and performance in school or college (as it did with Adam) or it might hinder their attempts to make friends or socialise. If, as a parent, you feel your child might have fears and worries that are beyond normal for their age range, it will be worth talking to teachers or learning mentors at their school to see if they've noticed anything relating to their learning, socialising or behaviour in general.

Children with anxiety have been seen to share many similar concerns as their peers, including worries about their schoolwork, friendships, personal harm and disasters. But where their experience of anxiety varies is in its intensity and how much it interferes in their lives. Children with anxiety are likely to experience more severe, chronic, and intense anxiety, which can be debilitating.

Changes in behaviour

You may have already noticed changes in your child's behaviour at home. Are they avoiding things they used to like doing? Are they moody, tearful or clingy? Are they spending more time on their own? From about 11 onwards it might be hard to distinguish symptoms of anxiety from normal teenage development – not every change in behaviour is down to an anxiety problem!

That said, if the changed behaviour turns into a pattern, or you just can't decide which is which, it will be worth asking questions of your child to discover how they're feeling and establish if anything is worrying them. You might get a negative response, but if your instinct tells you something is wrong, and isn't being said, keep trying. As we saw with Adam, an anxiety problem that goes undiagnosed and untreated often continues in various ways for years to come, affecting your child's life even into adulthood.

Remember: If your child does suffer from an anxiety problem it is unlikely to get better on its own without help.

How does worry and anxiety start?

As a parent or a teenager, you might ask yourself, 'How did these worries and anxieties start, and why?' It's an interesting question, but it's worth saying that we don't need an answer to treat them! That said, sometimes it's useful to know, especially if you're helping a child through a treatment approach like this one. Research suggests that it is a combination of several factors including genetics, family dynamics and / or external triggers. However, it is important to say that **no fault or blame on the part of a parent, child or caregiver should be attached to an episode of anxiety disorder**. We all have moments of anxiety; it is when they become frequent and life-affecting that we consider anxiety a problem.

Adam worried about his mum dying. As we have mentioned, this is a normal worry for children to have at some stage in their development. He looked up and saw a cloud, then thought that if he was the only one to see that cloud, his mum would die. So what is a normal worry in a child, that a parent might die, suddenly became an obsession, and a compulsion about looking at clouds develops from it. It's also normal for children to develop habits, but when these habits become something which causes distress if they are not done properly or completed, we can be pretty sure we might have a problem with anxiety, and in Adam's case, an obsessional problem that became OCD.

Life experiences can have a role to play in childhood anxiety, and disorders can develop after a traumatic event (such as encountering an angry dog) or there can be anxiety already in the family, which a child models their behaviour on. If a parent is nervous about spiders and does everything to avoid them, it's no surprise that their child might be the same. But again, **it doesn't always follow and no blame need be attached**, either by parent or child. And if you are a parent and you're anxious, it's really worth speaking to someone qualified about your anxiety, and how you might work through it in order to then help your child.

Chapter 6

Anxiety and Obsessional Disorders in Children

This chapter is about some of the most common anxiety and obsessional disorders seen in children and teenagers. You may recognise some of these behaviours in your child. Or if you're a teen, take a read through and see which ones might apply to you.

Again, let me stress that it is normal for all of us to have fears, worries, and anxieties. It is only when they become very distressing and interfere a lot in our lives that we can consider them to be symptoms of an anxiety problem.

We have provided a list of anxiety disorders for reference below. That said, children and young people develop quickly, so pinning them down to one diagnosis is not always easy, or indeed, helpful. It is also common for children who have problems with anxiety to meet the criteria for more than one anxiety disorder. So please view this as a general guide and if in doubt, do seek professional advice and help.

Common anxiety and obsessional disorders

Separation Anxiety Disorder. This is worries, fears, and anxieties around separation from parents, carers or other people to whom the child is attached. It can also be around places, usually the home. It is quite possible that Adam's first brush with anxiety was Separation Anxiety Disorder, although it was undiagnosed. Children will worry about people close to them dying or being harmed in some way, or think about something bad happening to them (getting lost, being kidnapped) which results in them being separated from a major attachment figure. Specific symptoms of this disorder are reluctance to leave home or go anywhere due to fear of separation, nightmares about separation, and refusal to sleep away from home, or go to sleep without the main caregiver at home. Worry around losing parents or caregivers is common in childhood; however, if it is causing real interference in the child's life and the symptoms last for more than four weeks, it's likely that it requires treatment.

Selective Mutism. This is an ongoing failure to speak in certain social occasions where the child would normally be expected to speak, for example, at school or family events. This problem will interfere with schooling and general communication with others, and while children might speak at home they will remain quiet in front of teachers, friends or relatives. This is a rare disorder and the onset is before the age of five years.

Specific Phobias. These are strong fears and anxieties about certain objects and situations (eg: dogs, spiders, heights, water, the dark, loud noises, strangers, aeroplanes, blood, vomit, etc.) A phobia will last for at least six months, and the fear is disproportionate to the danger posed by the object or the situation. For example, a person with a phobia around spiders will avoid going into a dark shed or garage for fear of seeing cobwebs and spiders.

Social Anxiety Disorder. This is a fear of embarrassing yourself in front of your peers. Up to 75 per cent of cases begin between the ages of eight and 15. For diagnosis as Social Anxiety Disorder, it must last for six months or more, and the fear of being embarrassed or ashamed will be out of proportion to the threat. Like all anxiety disorders, not treating it can cause significant difficulties in later life.

Generalised Anxiety Disorder. A person worries excessively about a range of different things, and feels they cannot control these worries. Children and adolescents tend to worry about school and sporting performance, punctuality, and catastrophic events. These worries can interfere with the child's or young person's ability to enjoy activities at home, at school, or with friends. Although it is not often diagnosed until adulthood, children and adolescents can have this disorder, and they are often referred to as 'worriers'.

Panic Disorder. When we worry about panic attacks re-occurring and go out of our way to avoid the possibility. As a reminder, panic attacks are intense feelings of anxiety which come on quickly and are extremely unpleasant. Panic disorder is less common in children, but may occur in adolescents.

Agoraphobia is a fear of being in a specific situation and not being able to escape or find help if the person has a panic attack, or some other embarrassing symptoms. These specific situations are using public transportation, being in open spaces (e.g. parking lots or markets) being in enclosed spaces (e.g. theatres or shops), standing in lines or being in a crowd, or being outside home on their own. Agoraphobia commonly begins in adolescence and it is often diagnosed alongside panic disorder.

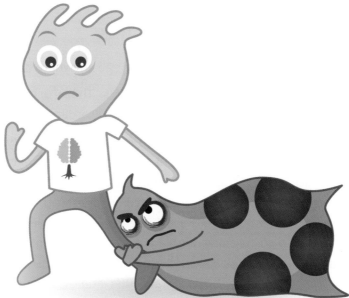

All anxiety disorders have a collection of anxiety symptoms, and common symptoms of anxiety in children and young people include:

- Intense feelings of anxiety
- Difficulty concentrating
- Irritability
- Unwillingness to take part in activities
- Refusing to speak
- Shrinking away from the situation
- Refusal to leave main caregiver or leave the home
- Freezing when the situation or object of fear is encountered
- Excessive clinginess
- Difficulty sleeping
- Tiredness
- Muscle aches
- Chest pains
- Crying
- Having tantrums
- Sweatiness
- Light-headedness
- Shaking

These are the main anxiety disorders that children and young people may experience, and you have probably noticed that many of the symptoms overlap. You may fit into one or more of these categories, but if you don't it doesn't mean you're not experiencing anxiety of some kind and it is not interfering in your life. As clinicians we treat these diagnoses as guides rather than a set of criteria that have to be religiously ticked off. In addition, children and young people may fit into more than one category at the same time. Again, it is common to cross over different diagnoses. For example, a fear of social situations may be classified as both social anxiety disorder and a specific phobia.

Obsessional disorders

This leads us on to **Obsessional Compulsive Disorders**. These used to be classified under 'Anxiety Disorders' but are now in a category of their own. Disorders in this category include:

Obsessive Compulsive Disorder (OCD). As we've read, Adam's anxiety developed into OCD and he suffered terribly from it. It is a problem defined by having excessive and unwanted obsessional thoughts which cause distress, and compulsions, rituals or other behaviours to try to stop or 'undo' the thoughts or prevent the feared outcome, or any other repetitive behaviour the person feels they have to do in response to these thoughts. For example, Adam's obsessions were about losing his mum, going mad, harming disabled people or old people, and strangling children, among others. His compulsions included excessive counting, handwashing, repeating words and phrases, avoiding people or situations, carrying handcuffs, and over-thinking the worry.

Body Dysmorphic Disorder (BDD). Here, a child or young person worries excessively about things in their appearance that are either not noticeable to others, or only appear to be slight or insignificant to others. The most common body areas people with BDD worry about are facial features and skin appearance, but it can be about any part of the body. The person goes to great lengths to disguise these 'problems', for example, using excessive make-up or wearing particular clothes to hide the perceived problem. The most common age for BDD to start is around 12 or 13, and two thirds of people with BDD develop it before they are 18. We do not cover BDD specifically in this book, but as explained, it has its roots in childhood and adolescence and can be a lifelong problem if left untreated.

Other Obsessional Disorders that can start in childhood and adolescence include **Hoarding**, which is when people find it difficult to get rid of things they don't need, and feel they must save. In young people this can start with small piles of rubbish or collections of insignificant things. There is also **Trichotillomania**, when a person pulls out their own hair, resulting in hair loss, and **Excoriation Disorder**, which involves compulsively picking at the skin.

So these are the anxiety and obsessive disorders we might find in children and young people. It's worth pointing out as we did before that one anxiety or obsessional problem can exist alongside others ('co-morbidity') so if you have one problem, you're quite likely to have others too. If this is the case please don't worry; it is not at all uncommon and our treatment method works across the board.

Depression

Also existing alongside anxiety is **Depression**. This is low mood which has lasted for more than two weeks, with symptoms including irritability, changes in appetite including loss of appetite or increased eating, insomnia or excessive sleeping, reluctance to socialise, lack of energy and motivation, and increased tearfulness.

Depression is often experienced alongside an anxiety or obsessional problem, and it makes sense given how much the problem can interfere in life. However, if you are worried that your child or teen is suffering from depression then we would recommend speaking to a professional for more help and guidance. While feeling low is normal, particularly as a teenager, depression is a more serious condition and can be harder for young people to see their way through. A proper assessment and diagnosis is vital and an evidence-based treatment approach can then be started. Your child may still be able to continue working through this book at the same time as receiving treatment for depression. Often the depression can reduce when the anxiety or obsessional problem resolves but it is still important to seek professional help if you think your child or teen is depressed.

Now that we've looked at the main anxiety and obsessional disorders in children and young people, we'll move on to examine how anxieties and obsessions work in the next chapter. And we'll see what people do to try and stop them, or push them away.

Chapter 7

The Truth About Anxiety

Let's look at bit more closely at anxiety to see how it works. Knowing and understanding this makes treating anxiety so much easier, so please read this chapter carefully and have a think about the questions at the end.

Thoughts, feelings and behaviour

First, we'll look at the link between **thoughts, feelings, and behaviour**, and how one is a **trigger** for another. We all have thoughts – if we didn't, we wouldn't be alive! We have thousands and thousands of thoughts every day. Some are sensible, practical, and useful, while others are silly, weird or random and seem to come from nowhere. **This is completely normal**. People without anxiety or obsessional disorders only pay attention to the thoughts they feel are useful, like remembering to buy a birthday card, or deciding which pair of shoes they'd rather buy. But for others, especially those with anxiety, their thoughts (even the silly ones) can trigger uncomfortable feelings and lead to the person behaving in certain ways to try to get rid of those thoughts and feelings, or try to stop the thought (now called a worry) from coming true.

Let's have an example. Two nine-year-old friends, Claire and James, are in the same class at school and have to make a presentation about someone famous on the same day. Claire is going to talk about her favourite athlete and thinks everyone will be interested in what she has to say. She feels positive and excited about the presentation and when she gives it, the class sits up and takes notice. Afterwards she is praised by the teacher for her confident manner.

James, on the other hand, is not looking forward to the presentation. He has chosen to talk about his favourite rugby player, but he thinks no one will be interested in him. That makes James feel nervous, sweaty, and anxious, and he thinks everyone will laugh at him and he'll blush. When it's his turn to stand up he makes an excuse that he feels ill and is sent to see the school nurse. He never makes the presentation and in years to come, is anxious about any kind of speaking in public.

Here we have two people in exactly the same situation, but both have very different responses.

Let's have another example. Katrina and Ellie are 12, and at a high school where the toilets aren't the cleanest. Both are worried about picking up germs from the handle on the toilet door and catching something. Katrina thinks, 'I don't really want to catch a cold or some other illness, but I could catch one anywhere. And I'm dying to use the toilet, so I might as well just open the door.' And she does.

Ellie, on the other hand, thinks, 'I don't want to catch a cold because I might pass it on to someone old, who might become really ill and even die. So even though I need the toilet, I daren't open the door.' And she doesn't, which leads her to worry about other things that could give her germs and illnesses. Plus she doesn't use the toilet and that is very uncomfortable too!

In both examples, do you see the link between their thoughts, their feelings, their bodily responses, and their behaviour? James thinks no one will be interested in his presentation, so he feels nervous and has a physiological response in his body – he becomes sweaty. His behaviour is to make an excuse that he is ill. Ellie thinks that if she catches a cold she will pass it on to someone vulnerable, so she feels anxious. Her behaviour is to avoid opening the door and using the toilet.

Our treatment approach explores the links between thoughts, feelings and behaviour and is based on a system called Cognitive Behavioural Therapy, or CBT for short.

What is CBT?

CBT is a way of looking at the things that happen to us in our lives, and helps us explore how we see them and what we do about them. CBT is the best treatment we have for anxiety and obsessional problems because it shows us how we respond to thoughts or events, and (if we have anxiety) how we can change those responses into ones that do not make us worried, anxious or afraid. Countless scientific studies have shown that CBT helps people to recover from anxiety and obsessional disorders, and that's why we have based our approach on it.

As we've seen above, no two people think about or respond to the same situation in exactly the same way. We can climb a steep rock face with no fear at all, but break down in tears when we find a small spider in our bedroom. Conversely, we can handle a tarantula without any worries, but feel sick and dizzy just standing at the bottom of the cliff. How we **think about** and **interpret** a situation is the key factor in how we **respond** to it. Do you remember we talked about the 'fight, flight or freeze' response to threats? When we're presented with a danger (or what we perceive to be a threat) our bodies respond by making us want to stand up to the threat, run away or freeze.

Younger children might have trouble saying exactly what it is that is making them anxious, whereas teenagers can usually be more specific. If you're a parent or caregiver of a younger child and you're having trouble with this, don't worry. That your child is feeling anxious about *something* is enough for you to be able to help them. Even if you can't quite tell what it is, you can gather that they are responding to a situation which feels threatening. You don't always need to figure it out exactly, because younger children's worries can jump around, as we saw in Adam's story.

Clues to problems

In children, avoiding something is a key sign that there is a problem. Because they can't always say exactly what is worrying them, younger children make excuses to avoid the situation. Headaches, stomach aches, and feeling sick are very common symptoms of anxiety and if you've gone through the standard checks to make sure there is nothing physically wrong with your child (i.e. no raised temperature, diarrhoea or actual vomiting) you can start to think about whether it is a response to a situation they find frightening and are worried about. They might also say that they don't want to go to school, or begin to ask repeated questions on the same topic to seek reassurance. Of course, this could pass very quickly without you having to do anything, but if it is going on for weeks you are best to intervene to try to help them understand and overcome the problem.

Tackling problems in a positive way

We will teach you how to do this later in the book, but for now let's look at some simple strategies you can use when your child has faced a fear positively. If your child has had worries about going to school, but has gone anyway, it is vital to follow that up with **positive reinforcement**. This is not reassurance that 'everything will be alright' (which is not always helpful, as we will see) but an acknowledgement that your child has made an effort to face their fear. Give a verbal reward by praising them, or physical rewards such as a treat, a cuddle, reading or playing a game with them; and be clear about what behaviour you are praising. All these rewards are a 'well done' for positive behaviour, and they should be applied as soon as possible after the event. Don't leave them too late – otherwise they lose their power!

We need to be able to support children's courage because sometimes taking these steps towards fear doesn't always go our way. The unpleasant thing they worry about might happen; they might get laughed at, or blush in front of the class. What is important is that they're rewarded for trying, because that way they will learn to try again, and eventually realise that things are never quite as bad as we think they will be.

What we discourage is responding unhelpfully to behaviours that we have identified as a problem. We want to encourage, not punish. I heard a story of a mother whose girls were anxious about going to school and refused to get changed into their uniforms. So she put them into the car and dropped them off in their pyjamas! That did nothing but reinforce their anxieties about school. Instead, she needed to tell them that although they were worried, worries are normal, and they were being brave by even getting out of bed and putting on their school uniforms. Ideally, they could have taken steps towards facing that fear together. Because, when you acknowledge the worries, you help to normalise them. Punishing just amplifies anxieties in the same way that if you kick a dog every time it doesn't retrieve the ball, you will end up with a highly-strung creature that will only respond to you out of their fear of being punished, not because they want to play 'fetch' with you.

Reassurance rights and wrongs

As we've mentioned above, it really isn't helpful if a child with anxiety seeks reassurance that 'everything will be alright', and then gets it. In fact, **reassurance reinforces anxiety and OCD**, and 'enough reassurance' is never enough. Seeking reassurance becomes a safety behaviour itself. That said, it is hard NOT to reassure someone that they will be okay, especially when it's your child in distress. But the less reassurance is given, the quicker you / your child will recover.

For example, if your child has worries over contamination and is anxious about some vegetables you've bought from the market, don't say, 'Yes, I'm sure they were all washed beforehand, and they don't have soil on them ...' Instead, say something like, 'I know you're worried about it, but as we've discussed, this isn't something we can fix or solve by talking about it.'

This isn't the easiest path to take but if it is done with kindness and understanding, it is the best approach by far. Family members can unwittingly collude in anxiety and OCD by reassuring, and if this is you, you need to ask yourself, 'Am I doing anything to feed into this, allowing it to grow?' If so, this is the point at which you need to stop complying with your child's requests.

If you're a teenager, you might be past expecting rewards from your parents or caregivers and value self-reliance more than constant pats on the back. However, pats on the back are no bad thing, and you are allowed to give yourself one now and again! It might help to think of a reward that you can give yourself after tackling fears or worries. It might be watching your favourite TV show, going to the cinema, buying those shoes you really want, or just spending time with friends. But it is important to recognise how courageous you have been in taking steps to overcome your problem.

Being kind to yourself

If you want to overcome your anxiety problem, you need to find the motivation to make some changes in your life. And, really importantly, you need to learn to be kind to yourself. To change, we have to take a journey that is non-judgemental and does not involve blame. We must be kind to ourselves during this journey. Anxiety makes it very easy to be self-critical and try to take the blame for everything. It's very easy to feel ashamed and embarrassed of having the problems we've described, but these kinds of feelings will hold you back from getting better.

Never forget - you are a deserving, worthwhile person. You deserve to be supported and treated with kindness. Treating yourself in a kind and non-judgemental way is incredibly important, and will really help kick-start your recovery.

To finish this chapter, here are a couple of checklists – one for you and one for your child – to help you focus on the sorts of anxiety or obsessional problems you or your child may be facing. At this stage it's not vital to 'nail down' exactly what the problem is, where it lies, or how it affects you. Just acknowledging that there is a problem is a good start. Have a look at the questions below and answer them honestly before moving on to the next chapter, which takes a specific look at the common problem of OCD in children and young people.

ANXIETY / OBSESSIONAL CHECKLIST FOR PARENTS AND CAREGIVERS

- Does your child have any sleep problems? (e.g. finding it hard to get to sleep, waking up in the night, feeling excessively tired in the morning)
- Does your child often seem irritable, on edge, or tearful?
- Does your child tend to be excessively clingy and seem unwilling to be parted from you or other loved ones, even for short periods? Does your child experience tearfulness / moodiness?
- Does your child try to avoid going to school?
- Has your child experienced changes in behaviour or started to avoid things they used to like?
- Is your child withdrawn or becoming isolated?
- Does your child have unpleasant thoughts, images, doubts or worries that repeatedly enter the mind?
- Does your child worry excessively about terrible things happening?
- Does your child do anything to avoid having these worries?
- Does your child have concerns about acting on an unwanted and senseless urge or impulse?
- Does your child feel driven to perform certain acts over and over again? (This may include checking, confessing, counting, examining their body for signs of illness or anxiety, touching things, repeating actions, collecting objects, arranging things, washing, and cleaning.)

ANXIETY / OBSESSIONAL CHECKLIST FOR CHILDREN

- Do you ever have strange or unpleasant thoughts, images, doubts or worries in your head?
- Do you worry a lot about terrible things happening?
- Do you do anything to avoid having these worries?
- Are you scared about acting on your unwanted feelings and urges?
- Do you do things over and over again to try and make yourself feel better, for example, checking, confessing, counting, examining your body for signs of illness or anxiety, touching things, repeating actions, collecting objects, arranging things, washing, and cleaning?
- Do you find it hard to get to sleep, or keep waking up in the night? Do you often feel tired when you get up in the morning?
- Do you feel more cranky and irritable?
- Are you more clingy around your family and loved ones? Do you want to stay with them instead of going out?
- Do you ever feel sad or moody?
- Do you ever try to avoid going to school?
- Do you think your behaviour has changed a lot? Maybe you're avoiding the things you used to like doing?
- Do you ever feel withdrawn and lonely?

Please note, these checklists are provided as guides and are not exhaustive lists of anxiety or obsessional symptoms that children experience. They are a starting point to think about how problems might manifest themselves in children and how we can start to help them overcome them.

Chapter 8

OCD in Children

In this chapter, we will look at **Obsessive-Compulsive Disorder (OCD)** in children in more detail. As we know, Adam's anxieties developed into OCD and he suffered from this well into adulthood. If he'd been given help and treatment at an earlier stage, his life would not have been so badly affected by anxiety and OCD.

I've mentioned that my definition of OCD is of an **obsessional problem** that can be about absolutely anything, resting on a bed of anxiety, depression, shame and guilt. It is marked by persistent, unwanted and disturbing thoughts, images, doubts, feelings and urges which we call intrusions, with the **compulsive** urge to get rid of these thoughts, images, doubts, feelings, and urges or doing 'something' about them to stop an awful consequence from happening, e.g. *'if I don't look at the clouds my mum won't die'*) or trying to make sure you don't feel that is your fault if something does happen.

Is OCD in children common?

OCD in children is not uncommon. It is estimated that between two and three per cent of children worldwide suffer from it and studies show that it is more common in adolescence than we previously thought. In a way this is good news because it means the signs of OCD are being spotted much more quickly now, so good treatment can begin much earlier. In fact, around 25 per cent of cases of OCD have started before the person is 14 years old.

It also means that you, as a parent of an OCD child, or someone who suffers from OCD, are not alone!

There is a much better understanding of OCD now, and plenty of support groups and charitable organisations that you can turn to for help. OCD is often marked by feelings of isolation (because the sufferer feels too ashamed or frightened to tell someone about their anxieties) but there is help out there. Reading this book is a great place to start.

Obsessions

What are **obsessions**? Well, as we saw in Adam's story, these are worries that can be about anything. His started with a simple worry about his mum dying and jumped around until they focused on thoughts of harming other people, which was very disturbing for him. We also call these obsessional thoughts '**intrusive thoughts**' (and images, doubts, feelings, and urges) and they are uncontrollable, seemingly popping into our head regardless of whether we want them or not, causing considerable distress.

As he says, Adam is the last person in the world who would harm someone. But he gave **importance** to an unwanted intrusive thought about harming people *('I must be a dangerous person if I'm having these bad thoughts')* and then he felt anxious, guilty and wrong for having such thoughts.

In other words, he took a silly thought too seriously.

In taking these intrusions too seriously, people then assume that they have to do something to stop the bad thing from happening (e.g. Adam's mum dying) or to stop having these types of thoughts altogether. This is when people develop compulsions or rituals, along with other safety behaviours (such as avoiding people or certain situations), to reduce this threat, or to try to stop having the intrusions in the first place. On their own these compulsions or rituals might seem a bit silly, such as turning a light switch on ten times. As we know, a ritual like that won't have any effect on whether a bad thing, such as someone dying, will happen or not. However, a person with OCD absolutely believes this compulsion, ritual or safety behaviour will actually stop the feared thing from happening.

This, in essence, is what OCD is all about: taking a thought, an image, doubt, feeling or urge that should never have been taken seriously in the first place but treating it very seriously, and then doing something about this thought to reduce the likelihood of the bad thing happening, or trying to stop yourself having these intrusions altogether. By doing this, you actually increase the likelihood of the intrusions happening. It's a bit like closing your eyes and being told not to think of a red fire engine, or a blue giraffe … and the first thing you do is think of the fire engine or the giraffe!

That said, for younger children and adolescents it can be very hard NOT to pay attention to unwanted thoughts, images, urges or doubts.

Describing worry

Some children might be able to talk about their worries. A six-year-old who stands in dog poo, who thinks that her hands are forever dirty and begins to wash them over and over again may be able to tell an adult why she feels unclean. Another child of the same age might have an unfocused worry about strangers, but can't explain this properly. Instead, he demands to see that all the doors and windows are locked, night after night. Adam was frightened that something would happen to his family. He couldn't or wouldn't tell anyone this; instead, he developed the 'four times' ritual (looking under his bed four times, turning the light on and off four times) that he felt would keep his family safe.

Even if they can't or won't tell you what is worrying them, it's highly likely your child is thinking along the lines of:

'If I don't do this (e.g. checking doors, counting etc.,) something bad will happen'

And / or

'Doing this means I won't have any awful thoughts or images etc.'

And / or

'Doing this (checking, counting etc.) makes me feel better.'

As a parent of a younger child, you are often likely to see the behavioural response (**compulsion, ritual or safety behaviour**) to the worry before you know the worry itself.

Challenging this behaviour

At this stage, it's important that you challenge the behaviour; not in a punishing way but as a means to find out where the worry lies. Intervening in these compulsions now will save you and your child a lot of heartache in the future. Adam was not so lucky; OCD just wasn't as widely understood when he was a child. But now, there is lots more information and support available, so do please use it.

To test how your child is feeling, it might be worth interrupting some of the compulsions to see how they react. If it's number-based (like Adam's 'four times' ritual) you might notice your child becomes irritable or angry when you interrupt them. If they have to repeat it, it's a clear sign that they believe they will 'have' to complete it in order to feel okay. That suggests it is an obsessional problem.

If your child is at school and you suspect they are carrying out rituals, it would be worth asking teachers or support staff if they've noticed any unusual behaviour. Adam's anxiety started when his mum left him at the school gate, and in younger children the worry underneath the behaviour could well be connected with going to school. One young person I worked with was worried about not doing well at school, and his OCD made him repetitively write all his classroom work in his book over and over again. This was something that the school noticed before his parents.

Other signs to look out for might be increased tiredness and lethargy, as a result of your child carrying out compulsions or rituals instead of going to sleep on time. You might also notice they are increasingly late leaving the house because they are spending so much time making checks before they go.

It is worth repeating that seemingly 'odd' behaviour is normal in children and young people, and it might just be a phase they will quickly grow out of. We only need to be concerned when it is significantly interfering in their life (this could be socially or academically, at home, or while taking part in sports or leisure activities) – and this is when we need to intervene.

You might ask, what's the difference between anxiety and OCD, and how can you tell which (if any) your child is suffering from? Both are based on fears and worries, but the responses can be quite different. **With anxiety, the responses might be:**

- Irritability
- Tearfulness
- Somatic complaints such as stomach ache or headache
- Avoiding friends or other social situations
- Reluctance to go to school
- Avoidance of specific things or situations
- Clinginess
- Withdrawal
- Moodiness

Whereas in OCD, the responses could include:
- Switching lights on and off
- Checking taps are off and windows are closed
- Excessive cleaning
- Excessive handwashing or showering
- Counting rituals
- Refusing to let go of old or apparently useless items
- Requests for family members to repeat phrases or answer the same question
- Eating food in a particular order
- Ordering items in a particular way

This is only a handful of OCD behaviours. Of course there is overlap between the responses to anxiety, worry, and OCD, and you are likely to see a child with OCD have both the compulsive ritualised responses and some of the more general anxiety responses listed above. But a child with anxiety problems (who doesn't have OCD) will not engage in these types of rituals. So what differentiates the two is that **in OCD the child believes that they may be responsible for something awful happening, or that they will never feel okay again**, unless they complete rituals or compulsions. Remember, OCD is about having intrusive thoughts, images, feelings or doubts, and worrying that these mean something bad or awful will happen, including never feeling 'okay' or normal (with an absence of anxiety responses) ever again. The child believes that they can make things 'safe' through compulsive behaviour. They may also feel that they have to do something to try and stop having intrusions, or 'undo' or cancel out the intrusion.

Worry is more about normal everyday events and situations, or about future things happening. Everyone worries – people with OCD are worriers, but not all worriers have OCD! It isn't the content of the worry that's important; it's what we do with the worry that counts, so worry only becomes a problem when it is excessive and causes interference in the child's life. While 'worriers' will also have safety behaviours to prevent the worry from happening, they are not ritualised as in OCD, and they don't feel compelled to do them.

The next section of this book will be aimed at younger children. We'll look at ways to help them to identify their worries and address them using our unique approach. We'll be using a variety of techniques and worksheets that parents (or caregivers) and children can understand and work on together. These will give you a better sense of anxiety, worry, and OCD, and how they interfere in our lives. Most importantly, we'll find ways to help you or your children start to get the better of them.

Part II
Managing Anxiety in Children

Chapter 9

Let's Meet Skeet

For parents and caregivers: In this section, we will introduce our method to help your child understand and manage their anxiety. Our CBT-based approach will help them to see the connections between their worries, how they feel and what they're doing (or not doing) to make them go away. This advice will be helpful for children with OCD too - and there'll be a dedicated section for them later on.

Please take time to read the information with your child. We know that even young children can engage with the concepts of CBT if they are presented in a way that is clear and engaging.

Hi! This section of the book is all about YOU!

So, who are you?

We know you have some worries and anxieties, but there's more to you than that.

So tell us more ...

My name is: _____

I am _____ years old

I live with: _____

My hobbies (or things that I like doing) include: _____

When I'm at school I like: _____

I am working through this book because:

_____

_____

_____

_____

Okay, now we know a bit more about you, let's find out about your worries ...

What are worries?

Worries are thoughts, or ideas, or doubts, or nagging little things in our head which tell us that something will not be okay in the future, or may be about something bad that has happened.

Are you feeling worried? What are you worried about?

How do you feel when you worry?

We all have worries, even Skeet. This is Skeet.

Skeet is an ordinary kid, just like you.

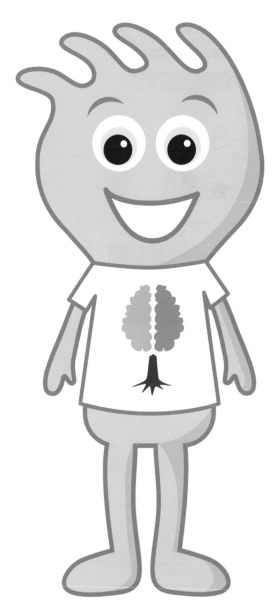

Most of the time, Skeet feels happy with his life.

He likes going to the park to play with his football.

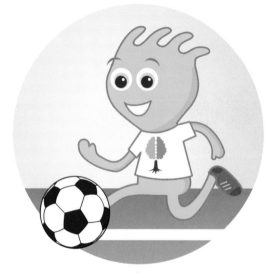

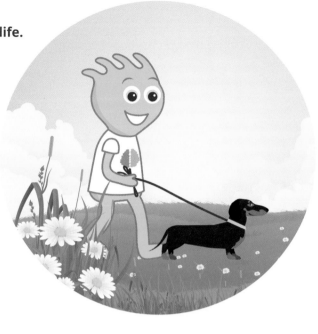

And walking his dog.

He absolutely loves getting presents.

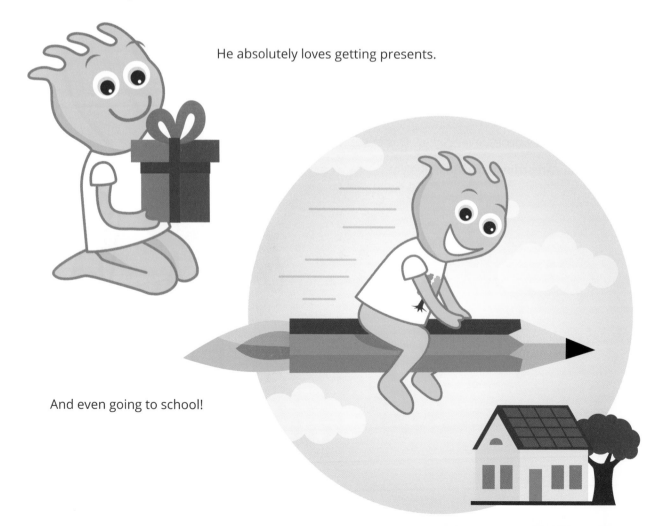

And even going to school!

He worries about thunderstorms.

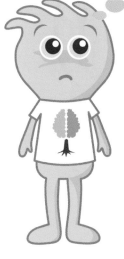

And about snakes
(even though he's never seen one).

**He worries that no one will
choose him for the school team.**

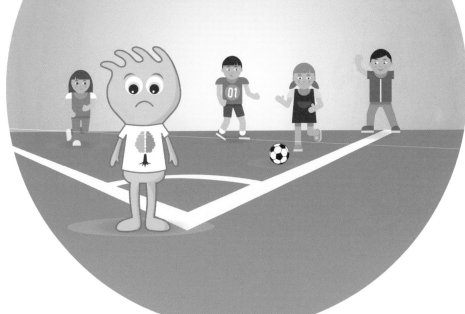

But sometimes, Skeet worries about things.

Sometimes he's not sure what he's worrying about. He just feels 'funny'.

We all have worries.

Even those kids who seem really confident worry about things.

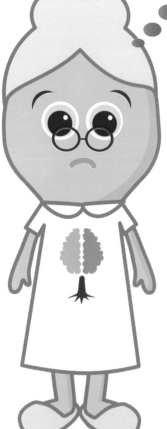

Oh dear, where could Tiddles be?

Even grown-ups worry!

Worry is a very normal part of being human. In fact, it started way back in the days of the cavemen, who were hunted by some very fierce animals that wanted to eat them! When they saw one of these animals coming they either chose to fight:

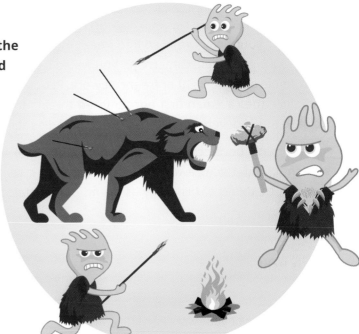

Or they 'took flight':

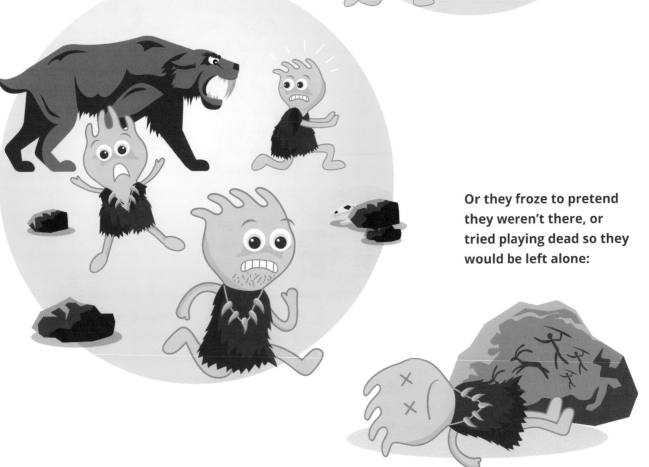

Or they froze to pretend they weren't there, or tried playing dead so they would be left alone:

This is called 'fight, flight or freeze' and it is the normal way people react to our worries. If something unexpected happens and it gives you a 'funny feeling' in your body ...

Imagine if an aggressive alien appeared in front of you. My reaction would be to run very fast! But maybe your body would go into freeze mode – maybe you'd stay still like a statue so that the alien would ignore you. Or perhaps, you would feel brave and you'd want to fight that alien. This is an example of 'fight, flight or freeze' at work. People have had these feelings for millions of years, ever since the cavemen first encountered threats to their survival. It's funny because although we're so much cleverer than they were, our bodies still react to scary events in just the same way.

Worry only becomes a problem when it won't go away. It's a bit like an annoying itch: you scratch it, and it goes away for a bit – but then it comes back again later. When this happens to Skeet, he thinks of his worry as a kind of monster. So guess what Skeet has called his worry monster …

This is Itch!

You try hard, but your worry won't go away.

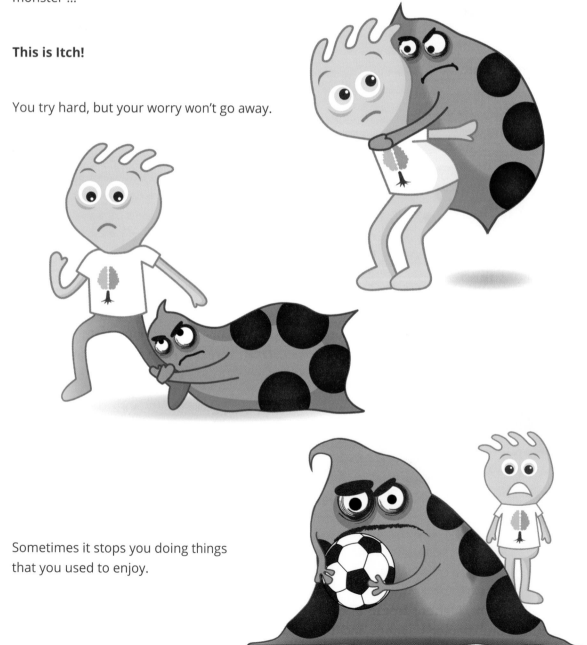

Sometimes it stops you doing things that you used to enjoy.

Or it makes you feel silly and embarrassed.

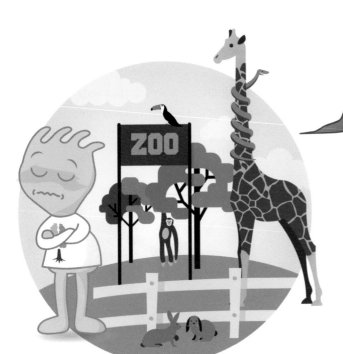

Or it makes you stop going to places you used to like visiting.

Sometimes all the worries come along at once.

And that makes you feel very worried, very sad, very afraid, and very tired.

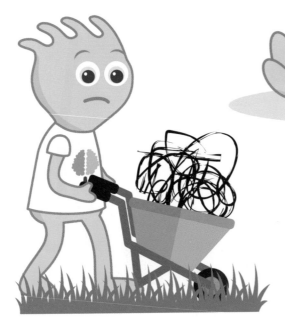

Having worries is like filling up a wheelbarrow. You put one thing in it, and while it's a little bit heavy, you can still push it around, or tip it out easily.

But if it's full of things, it becomes very heavy, hard to push around and not easy to tip out. Having lots of worries is hard to deal with. It's not nice carrying them all around with us, and we don't know how to get rid of them.

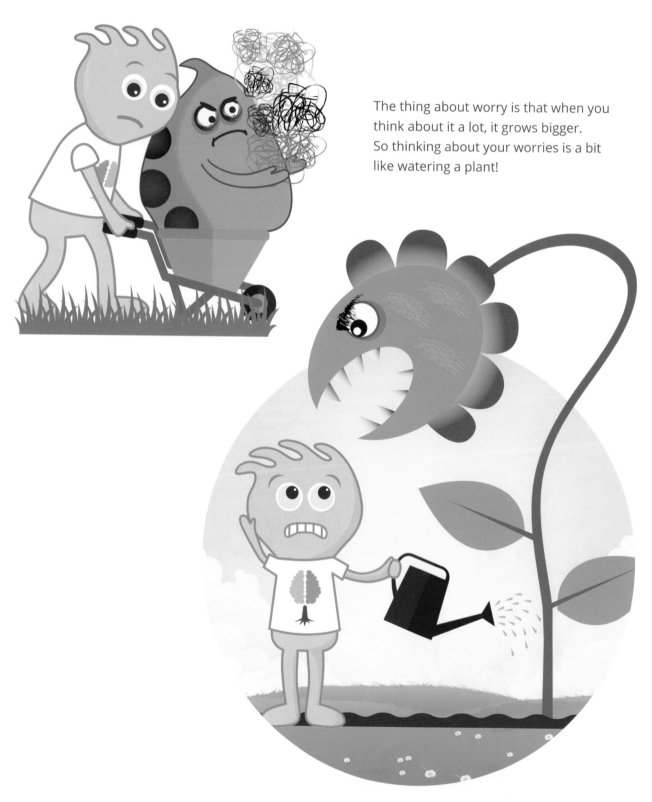

The thing about worry is that when you think about it a lot, it grows bigger. So thinking about your worries is a bit like watering a plant!

So – what are your worries? You might find it helpful to write them down in the box below.

These are my worries:

What are feelings?

We've said how worry makes us 'feel'. But what do we mean when we talk about 'feelings'? What are 'feelings'?

Feelings describe how we feel, or the reaction we have when something happens to us. When it's your birthday, and you get the present you've always wanted, you feel happy. If someone takes that present away, you might feel angry. If you played with it just once, then accidentally broke it, you would feel sad. If your younger sister or brother broke it, you would feel annoyed. We also call these feelings 'emotions'. As well as 'happy', 'sad' and 'angry' we could add 'worried', 'confused' 'stressed', 'ashamed', and 'embarrassed', and many more different types of feelings.

Here are some faces. You will notice they all have different expressions. Have a look at each face and see if you can guess the correct feeling or emotion each face is showing by matching it with the words under the picture.

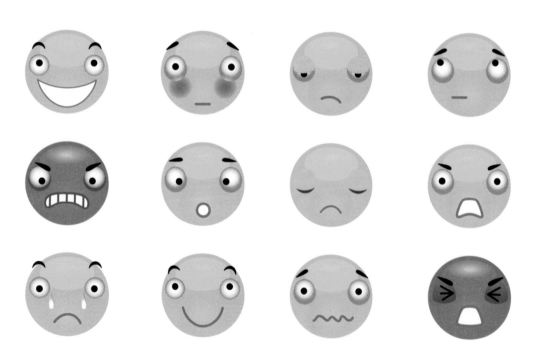

- Ashamed
- Sad
- Joyful
- Angry

- Stressed
- Upset
- Embarrassed
- Lonely

- Confused
- Worried
- Happy
- Annoyed

These are all types of feelings. Have you had any of these feelings lately? If so, pick three and put them in the box below. You might find it helpful to say why you felt that way.

I felt   because: _____

_____

_____

I felt   because: _____

_____

_____

I felt   because: _____

_____

_____

Okay, now we know what feelings and emotions are, let's have a look at how our worries make us feel. Remember the cavemen? Remember they had to choose to fight the sabre-toothed tiger, run away from it, or pretend not to be there? They didn't have much time to think about it, because the tiger was coming to eat them!

There aren't any sabre-toothed tigers around today, thank goodness! But there are other things that make us worried or anxious. If we hear a police car or fire engine going past with its siren on, how do we feel?

Scared? Happy? Sad? Lonely?

The answer, of course, is 'scared'. Even if it's only a little bit scared, we still put our hands over our ears to keep out the noise and we look up to see where it is coming from – a bit like a rabbit in a field when it senses danger!

What's happening in my body?

What else do we feel when we worry about something? As well as feeling 'sad' or 'lonely' or 'frightened', we also have sensations inside our bodies too.

We might notice ...

Like we have butterflies in our tummy.

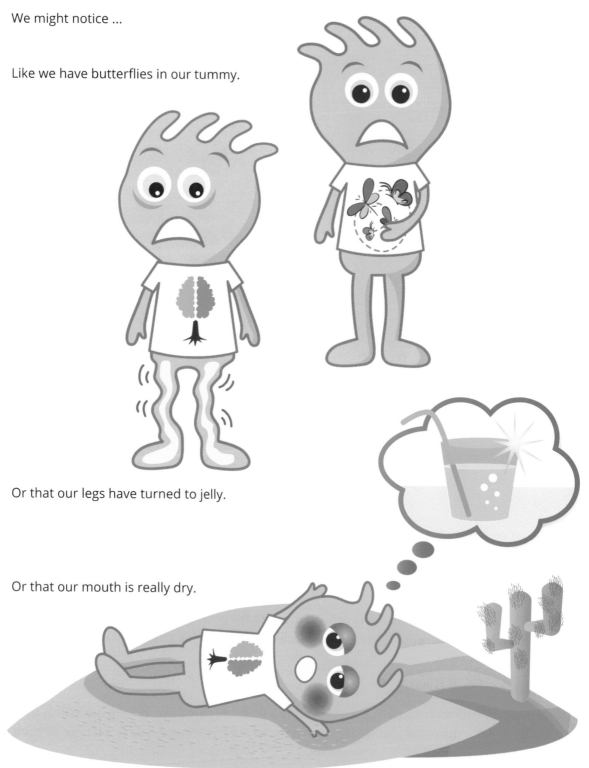

Or that our legs have turned to jelly.

Or that our mouth is really dry.

Have a look at the words below, and see if you recognise any of these things happening to you when you feel worried:

Breathless
Tummy ache
'Butterflies' in the tummy
Tingly
Heart beating quickly
Jelly legs
Shivering
Dizzy
Feeling sick

To help you, here's a picture of Skeet with these things happening to him. Have a look, and circle the ones you recognise.

Now, you might find it helpful to draw a picture of yourself in the box below and put a circle around the parts of your body that feel funny when you worry.

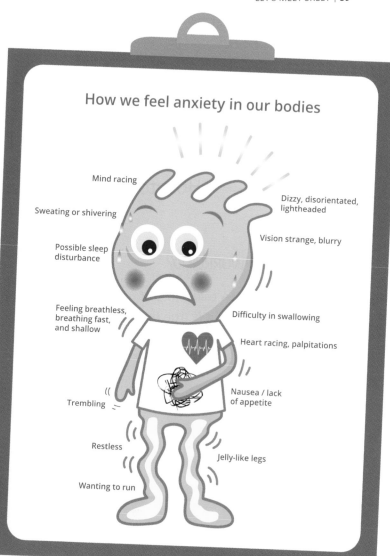

How we feel anxiety in our bodies

Mind racing

Sweating or shivering

Dizzy, disorientated, lightheaded

Vision strange, blurry

Possible sleep disturbance

Feeling breathless, breathing fast, and shallow

Difficulty in swallowing

Heart racing, palpitations

Trembling

Nausea / lack of appetite

Restless

Jelly-like legs

Wanting to run

Chapter 10

How to Deal with Your Worries

Can you stop worrying?

You've probably been told – lots of times, maybe – to 'stop worrying' because your worries are 'all in your head'. Well, it is true that worries are just thoughts that have become stuck, but that doesn't mean they don't feel 'real'. To you, they've become part of your life. Like Skeet, you feel that your worry is always around.

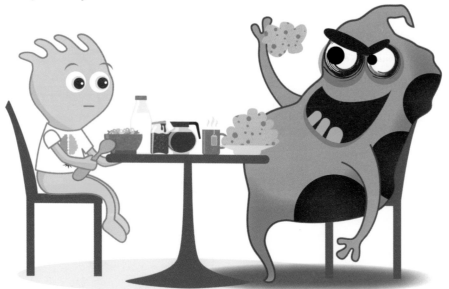

And no matter what you do, it's very hard to get rid of your worry. It hangs around with you all day, like a black cloud over your head, or like someone you don't want to spend time with. If one of your friends is being annoying, you might say to them, 'I don't want to play with you today', and hopefully they'd go away.

But the problem with worry is that it likes to stick around.

And no matter how hard you try, it can be very hard to shake off a feeling of worry.

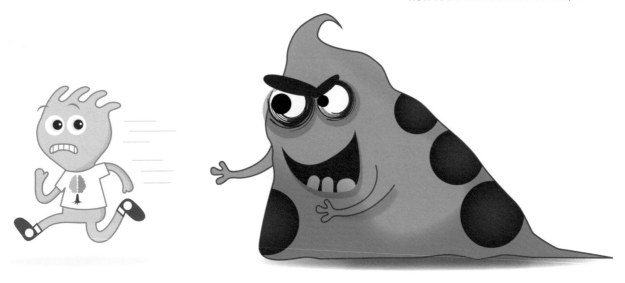

People try all sorts of ways to get rid of their worries. They might try not to think about them. This can work well for a short time, but it's a bit like someone telling you: 'Whatever you do, don't think of a blue giraffe... ' And what's the first thing you do? Write down your answer below ...

'When I'm told NOT to think of a blue giraffe, the first thing I do is ...'

That's correct! You think of a blue giraffe!

You might also avoid people and places (and even stop doing things you like doing) because they remind you of your worry. For example, Skeet is scared of snakes, so when his mum asks him if he'd like to go to the zoo with his friends, he says 'no' in case he sees a snake. It's a real shame, because normally, Skeet would love a trip to the zoo with his friends.

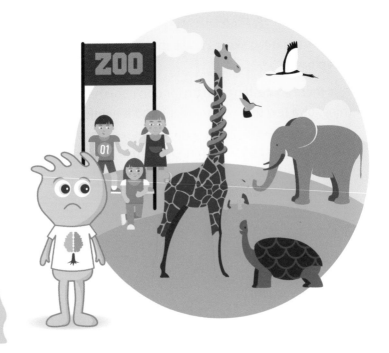

Skeet is also afraid of thunderstorms. So when the sky goes a bit cloudy and dark, Skeet feels funny. Normally this isn't a problem, he can stay inside. But if it happens before a games lesson at school, it gives Skeet a big problem. His teachers don't know why he's trying to get out of his games lesson, so they just think he's being naughty. But really, he's scared.

Having worries sometimes makes life difficult for Skeet. He misses out on having fun, and people think he's being a pain when he doesn't want to do something. Trying to get rid of his worries makes him feel better for a bit – but it doesn't really work properly.

Other kids who have worries like Skeet can worry about bad things happening that might be their fault, or have strange and unpleasant thoughts or pictures pop in their heads. These kids sometimes say special words, count in numbers or have 'lucky' things (clothes, toys and other objects) to help them get rid of their worries. When they say the special words, count the numbers or touch their lucky objects, they feel better. This is called OCD ('Obsessive Compulsive Disorder'). It's how we describe these types of worries that make us do things to try and get rid of them. But whatever we do, those worries just keep coming back!

We're going to talk more about OCD later, but for now, let's just say that it's very normal to try to make the worries go away!

Unfortunately, Skeet knows that it doesn't seem to matter what you do – your worries always creep back.

Is there something you do (or don't do) that makes your worries go away for a bit? If you do one thing, or a few things, you might find it helpful to write them down in the box below.

When I worry, this is what I do to make my worry go away ...

_____

_____

_____

_____

Okay, now you've remembered what you do (or don't do) to get rid of your worries, can you remember when you missed out on something, or someone got angry, **because** of your worries? You might find it helpful to write it down in the box below and say how it made you feel. If you want, you can draw a picture.

This is what happened when I worried ...

_____

_____

_____

_____

Do you ever wonder what other people worry about? We all have worries, and we're all worrying about something, but maybe not all the time.

What do other people worry about?

To see what other people are worrying about, pick three people from this list and try to think what they might worry about. If you want, you can ask them too!

Mum . . . .

Dad . . . .

Friend . . . .

Grandparent . . . .

Teacher . . . .

Neighbour . . . .

Brother . . . .

Sister . . . .

Aunt . . . .

Uncle . . . .

When you've thought about it, or asked them, you might find it helpful to write their answers down here.

My _____ worries about: _____

_____

My _____ worries about: _____

_____

My _____ worries about: _____

_____

You might be very surprised by their answers!

Like we said at the start, it is easy to tell someone to 'stop worrying' but quite hard to do – even for grown-ups. BUT – sometimes it's good to be brave, and do something that you're worried about. Why? Well, let's just say that Worry has a big secret – and when you know this secret, it might just change the way you think about your worries ...

Worry's Big Secret

Pssstttt!!! Shall we tell you Worry's secret?? The secret is that if you're brave, and you do something, even though you're worried about it, your WORRY BECOMES SMALLER AND SMALLER AND SMALLER each time you do the thing you're worried about! So if you're scared of spiders, I bet you think you couldn't ever touch one. But, if you can do it once, it will feel a little bit easier the next time. And it will keep on getting easier, every time you do it. I promise!

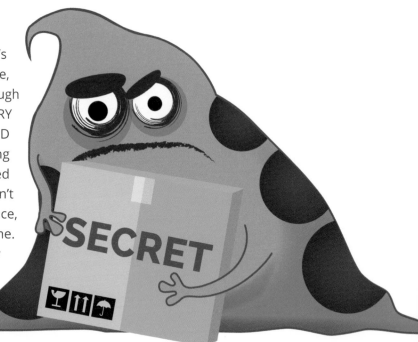

Isn't that a great secret to know? Even Skeet doesn't know it yet.

Before we go, let's tell you about George ...

George is nine, and his biggest worry is that the kids in his class will laugh at him if he answers a question from the teacher. He daren't put his hand up, and when she asks him to speak, he goes bright red and puts his head in his hands. The thing is, George is a clever boy and if he answered the question, he'd probably get it right. And no one would laugh at him!

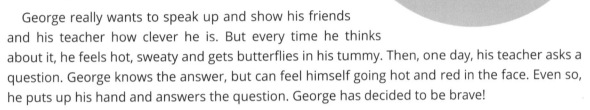

George really wants to speak up and show his friends and his teacher how clever he is. But every time he thinks about it, he feels hot, sweaty and gets butterflies in his tummy. Then, one day, his teacher asks a question. George knows the answer, but can feel himself going hot and red in the face. Even so, he puts up his hand and answers the question. George has decided to be brave!

'Well done, George,' says his teacher. 'Not only did you get the question right, I'm very pleased that you put up your hand and answered it.'

From that day on, every time George answers a question he notices his worry shrinking, bit by bit. Eventually, George will make his worry disappear altogether – because he was brave.

So let's share another secret ...

YOU can be brave too.

By being brave, YOU can make your worry shrink. Have a think about how you might do this. You might find it helpful to write your ideas in the box below:

To make my worry shrink I need to be brave and do ...

_____

_____

_____

_____

_____

_____

_____

Chapter 11

Thinking Traps and Other Ways to Beat Worry

Let's get clever

We've talked about how worry can stop you doing the things you enjoy, and how being brave can help to shrink worry down to size. The thing is, worry can be sneaky. Just when you think you've stopped one worry, another one can pop up – a bit like the fairground game where you have to 'Splat the Rat' when it pops up in different holes.

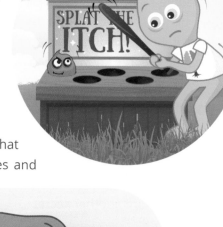

So - we need to be cleverer than worry. And the good news is, we can easily outsmart worry if we try!

Worry likes to lead us into what we call **'thinking traps'**. That means we get stuck in the way we think about our worries and can't get out of the trap.

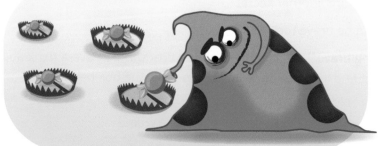

What are thinking traps?

For example, quite often we worry about things that might happen in the future, even though these things might not happen. And we also worry about things that have happened once (a thunderstorm, for example) but might not happen again for a while.

Disaster Thinking Trap

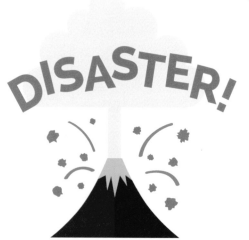

We think the worst is going to happen, and that everything will be a ... **Disaster. The thing about 'Disaster Thinking' is that the disaster you're worrying about very rarely comes true.**

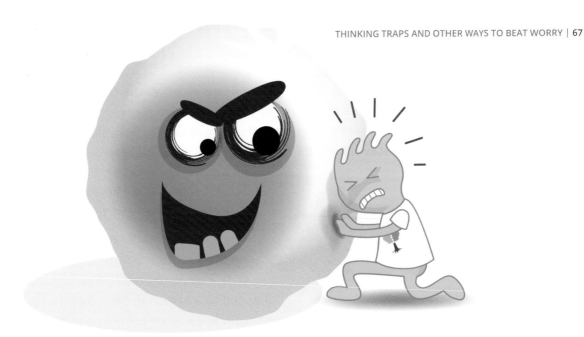

Snowballing Thinking Trap

Another trap that worry likes to set is called **'Snowballing'**. If you've ever played in the snow, you'll know that if you roll a small snowball across a field of snow, it will grow bigger and bigger as it picks up more snow.

So let's say you're learning to ride a bike, but you're worrying about falling off. Because if you fall off you might:

- Hurt yourself
- See other kids laughing at you
- Damage your bike
- Be too scared to get back on
- Worry about never learning to ride
- Worry that you'll be left out by your friends
- Worry that something is wrong with you

So you see how your worry has snowballed from something small into a Great Big Thing!

The thing about Snowball Thinking is that even IF the first worry comes true, it doesn't mean that all the other worries will come true as well!

Just Right Thinking Trap

Next there is the **'Just Right'** trap. You only stop worrying when you feel 'just right' and you think you have to feel 'just right' all the time.

Right?

WRONG!!

All of us – grown-ups and children – spend a lot of time trying to feel 'just right'. We do everything we can not to feel 'wrong'. Even if we feel angry, we try to be nice. Even if we feel sad, we try to look happy. Even if we feel frustrated, we try to remain calm.

The thing about Just Right Thinking is that trying to feel 'just right' all the time is very, very tiring and you can't make it last!. It's better to let yourself feel angry, sad, upset, lonely, and all the rest. They are all normal feelings even if they are uncomfortable – and if you don't fight them and let them stay for a little while they pass away quickly!

The Fortune Telling and Making Deals with Worry Thinking Traps

Next up we have **'Fortune Telling'**. Do you know what a fortune teller does? Well, they try to predict what is going to happen to a person in the future. But they don't really know what will happen – they just make clever guesses.

Sometimes we worry about the future because we think we can predict it. Jayne is ten and whenever she goes out with her parents, she thinks they will never find their way home again. This gives her a funny feeling in her tummy, and even when they DO get home safely, she still thinks that they will get lost one day.

The thing about Fortune Telling is that you can never know exactly what will happen in the future. You're worrying about something that hasn't happened, and probably never will. And even if it does happen, worrying about it won't change it!

When I was young, I used to worry that my cat would get run over, so I would try and do little deals with my worry. I'd say, 'Please keep my cat safe and I'll tidy my room every day.' But worry isn't a person and you can't do deals with it.

Magical Thinking Trap

Another thinking trap is **'Magical Thinking'**. This is when you do something (like counting or saying words) to stop something bad from happening. Jack's granny was in hospital, and Jack thought that if he counted to ten every two hours, she wouldn't die. It's very nice of Jack to be so concerned about his granny, but counting to ten won't make her better. Only doctors and nurses can do that!

The thing about Magical Thinking is that you can't change things from happening by making a spell. Have you heard of superstitions? Some people believe the superstition that walking under ladders will make something unlucky happen. So they always avoid walking under ladders because they think it will stop unlucky things happening to them. But what do you think would happen if you walked under a ladder? Do you think something unlucky would happen? Why don't you try it the next time you see a ladder? ...

Now we know what worry traps are, how do we make sure

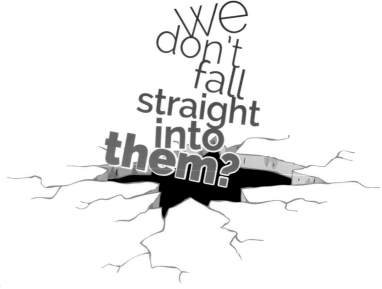

we don't fall straight into them?

Think good things instead.

Well, let's try something different – instead of thinking about bad things that might happen, try thinking about good things instead. Remember Jayne, who is frightened of getting lost? Imagine she's out on her bicycle, and let's see what happens …

First, she's gone to call for her friend Skeet.

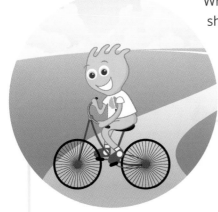

Where should they cycle to next? To the ice-cream parlour? To the shopping mall? To the swimming pool, or the beach? Tell you what – why don't you decide!? Choose where Skeet and Jayne should go, and then draw a picture, or write about what they did when they got there in the box below. You can make it as exciting, eventful and fun as you like!

Jayne and Skeet's great day out

Okay, so Jayne and Skeet have had their big adventure and now they're ready to go home. But wait? Do they know the way back? Isn't this Jayne's biggest worry coming true?

Let's pretend that they DO get lost, but let's also pretend that they have another exciting adventure before they find the road back to Jayne's house. In the box below, you might find it helpful to draw or write about what happens to them while they are lost.

Jayne and Skeet's getting lost adventure

Here are Jayne and Skeet arriving home safely after their adventures.

Did they have a good time? Yes – in fact they had an awesome time!

And do you know why they had such a good time, even though they got lost on the way home? **Jayne and Skeet are very sensible, clever children who know what to do in an emergency. They know that if they ever get really lost, they can find a police officer, make a phone call, or even get help from a shop. So this time, when they did get a bit lost, they didn't panic. Instead, they were able to enjoy all the good things that did happen, instead of worrying about all the bad things that didn't happen!**

Isn't that great? You expect something bad to happen because you've worried about it and instead, lots of interesting things happen!

So now it's your turn! I want you to draw a picture of yourself setting off on an adventure of your own. You can choose any form of transport you like: maybe a bike, a hot air balloon or even a space rocket!

Imagine you're going to do something that you'd like to do, if you could take your worry away. For example, if you like exciting funfair rides, but worry about getting separated from your mum and dad, imagine going to a busy theme park together.

Then, look at the questions below and say what happens.

How I felt on my adventure

My worry is ...

_____

Before I set off on my adventure, I felt ...

_____

_____

On the journey, these things happened ...

_____

_____

_____

When I experienced my worry I felt ...

_____

_____

_____

On the way home, these things happened ...

_____

_____

_____

A new story

So ... did you have an interesting time? Was it better than you expected? Did your worry bother you? If it didn't, or if it bothered you less than you thought it would, let's work out why ...

Without knowing it, you've created **A NEW STORY** about your worry. One that doesn't worry you, and actually makes you feel happy and excited!

We can all create **a new story** about our worry. The one we tell ourselves – about the thing that worries us, that makes us frightened and stops us from enjoying life – doesn't have to last forever. If you want, you can change the ending to make it different to the one your worry wants you to believe will happen. Remember when Skeet didn't want to go to the zoo because he was frightened of snakes? Let's pretend Skeet did go to the zoo (even though there are snakes there) and, in the box below, you might find it helpful to write a happy ending to Skeet's story about his day out.

Skeet's Day Out - happy ending by me!

_____

_____

_____

_____

_____

_____

_____

Ignoring worry

Another way to make your worry shrink is to ignore it.

It's not always easy to ignore a worry (especially when people say, 'just ignore it, and it will go away'!) but worries are a bit like plants. If you 'feed' and water them they will grow bigger.

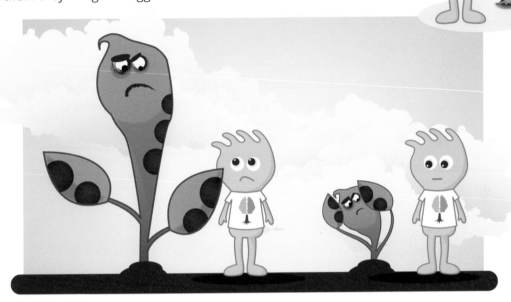

But if you don't think about them they shrivel up.

So even if we feel funny, we can ignore worries. Let's think about what you **could** be doing instead of worrying ...

You could be riding your bike. You could be playing sport. You could be reading a book, or watching TV.

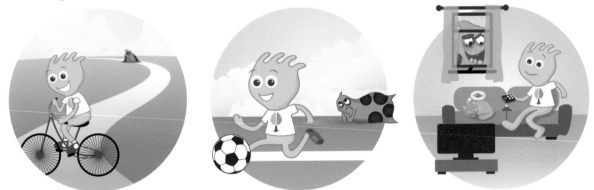

You could be doing anything that you **LIKE!** And 'like' is the right word, because worry stops you from doing things that you like. So don't let it! We know that isn't always easy, and even when you try to ignore worries they sometimes pop back into your head. That's okay – like Itch, they keep trying to hang around and annoy you – so just keep ignoring them, and don't worry if they come back now and again. One day, they'll get the message and leave you alone.

Below, think about, write down or draw what you would like to do instead of worrying. Then try and do that, and perhaps write down how it felt.

Instead of worrying, I'd like to ...

_____

_____

_____

_____

and when I did it, it felt ...

_____

_____

_____

_____

The Worry Bus

One other way we can try to manage our worries is by putting them on a **Worry Bus**. This isn't a real bus, but I know you're clever enough to imagine it! The Worry Bus picks up all your worries and keeps them on the bus for five minutes while you – you're the driver – listen to what they've got to say. Then, after five minutes, drop them all off at the next stop. Your bus will be nice and quiet again!

If you prefer, your mum or dad can drive the bus for you. Below, you can draw yourself, or your mum and dad, and all your worries on the bus.

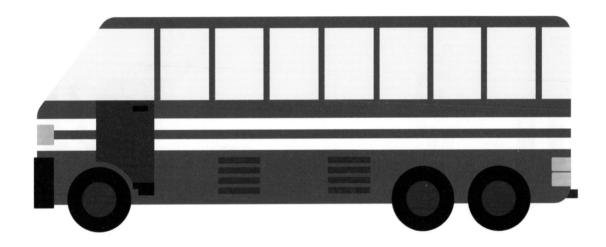

How did you get on? Try to do this for just five minutes each day and set an alarm so you know exactly how long you've got – but don't let the worry passengers get on the bus again once their five minutes has finished. And don't let them sneak on early either!

Like we said at the start of this chapter, worries are clever. But you are cleverer! Try all these little tricks and you'll outsmart worry – no problem!

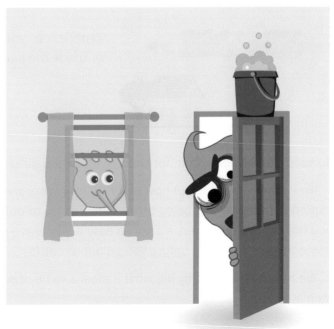

Being brave!

In the last chapters we've talked a bit about being 'brave'. You've probably done a lot of brave things in your life already, without even thinking that you were being brave.

You might have:

Been to the doctor's for an injection.

Been to the dentist for a filling.

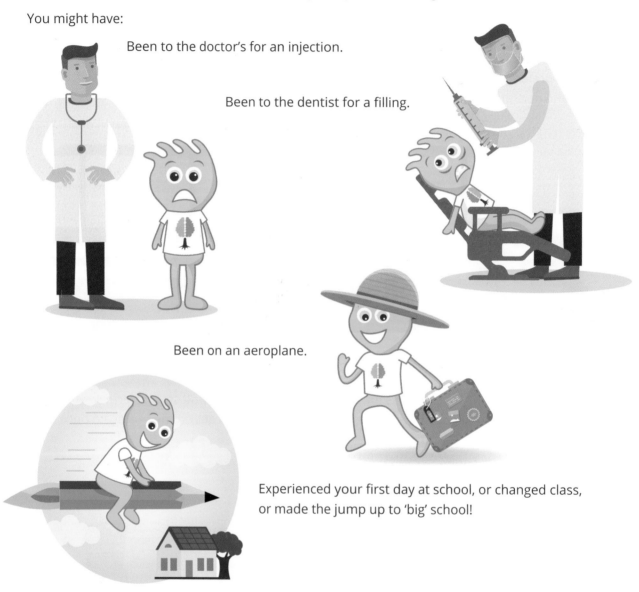

Been on an aeroplane.

Experienced your first day at school, or changed class, or made the jump up to 'big' school!

So even though you might not know it, bravery is already inside you!

Now we need to find out how to use that bravery and send Worry away! In the last chapter, we explored a few ways of being brave, standing up to our worries, and making them shrink. But as you might have found out, it's not so easy being brave just like that. Like a knight, you need to do some training exercises before you go out to battle.

We have to learn, bit by bit, what it means to be brave. And the best way to do it is to take one step at a time.

Be a scientist!

Science is about understanding how our planet and people work. We're sure you already know that people who study science are called scientists, and they do many experiments (or tests) to see if they can find out new things about the world, and about us. Scientists do this a lot, but they don't always get it right first time. Like a scientist, you are also experimenting with your Worry, testing it out to see what happens.

Woop!

If it doesn't go right, the scientist doesn't give up. Instead, he or she has another try, and another and another and another. Until finally ...

They get it right!!!

This is how some of our most amazing inventions have happened: by trying, failing, trying again, and eventually succeeding.

So keep trying! You might find it hard at first, but when you succeed you will feel ...

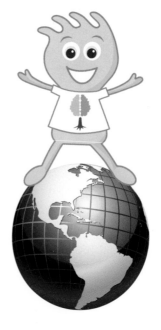

On top of the world!!

My worry ladder

Let's get you thinking like a scientist. But first, you're going to need to make yourself a worry ladder so you can take steps towards beating your worry.

Skeet has a worry ladder to help him deal with his fear of snakes. At the moment, Skeet is at the bottom of his ladder. To face his fear of snakes and conquer it, he needs to climb up the ladder, one step up at a time. Each rung of the ladder is a step closer to overcoming Skeet's fear.

Each step on the ladder is something that will help Skeet (and you) feel better about a worry. For example, Skeet could get a book from the library about snakes. He might feel a bit worried when he looks at the pictures, but he knows the snakes on the page won't hurt him. As he looks at the pictures his tummy might turn over. He might even get 'jelly legs'! But Skeet is trying to be brave, so he keeps looking at the pictures anyway. After he's flicked through the book a few times, Skeet feels a little bit better. Well done, Skeet! Take one step up the ladder!

Pick up a snake

Touch a snake in the pet shop

Look at the snakes in a pet shop

Go the to zoo, even though they have snakes

Look at a book about snakes

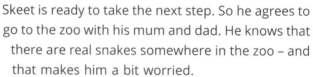

Skeet is ready to take the next step. So he agrees to go to the zoo with his mum and dad. He knows that there are real snakes somewhere in the zoo – and that makes him a bit worried.

But he knows he doesn't have to go into the Snake House if he doesn't want to. So, brave Skeet decides he can go to the zoo.

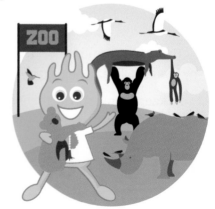

Skeet knew he would feel funny when he went to the zoo, but did it anyway. He was very brave. And here's a big secret about bravery ...

You might think that brave people don't get scared. But they really do. Being brave is all about being scared, but still doing the thing you need to do anyway. And then the more you do it, the less scary it gets. So all those funny feelings and jelly legs can be a good sign that you're actually being really brave.

Next, Skeet decided to go to a pet shop with snakes in tanks. Just before he goes through the door he feels a bit sick and his mouth goes dry, but because he's brave, he chooses to go in. From a distance, he looks at the snakes. Most look like they're asleep! Well done again, Skeet! Take another step up the Worry Ladder!

A few days later, Skeet's dad takes him for a walk in the countryside. Skeet's dad knows there are harmless snakes in the rocks, so they go looking for them. They spy one on a rock and it's asleep, so they creep right up to it and spend a few minutes looking at it. Even though he's very near to it, Skeet is only a little bit worried. Instead, he admires the snake's patterned skin. Skeet and his dad creep away without disturbing the snake.

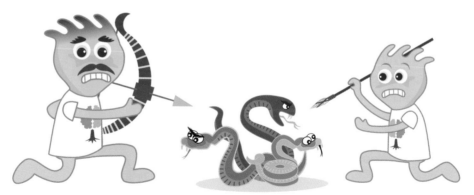

Next, Skeet's dad asks him if he'd like to visit the pet shop and maybe handle the snakes. Skeet feels funny about this, but he decides to go along. The pet shop owner takes out a snake and lets Dad hold it. Then, very gently, Skeet touches it.

'Dad,' says Skeet, 'do you think the shopkeeper will let me handle the snake?' 'Why don't we ask her?' replies Skeet's dad. The lady in the shop says it's fine, and although Skeet is really nervous, he picks up the snake and lets it move around his arm. By now, Skeet knows that every time he does something

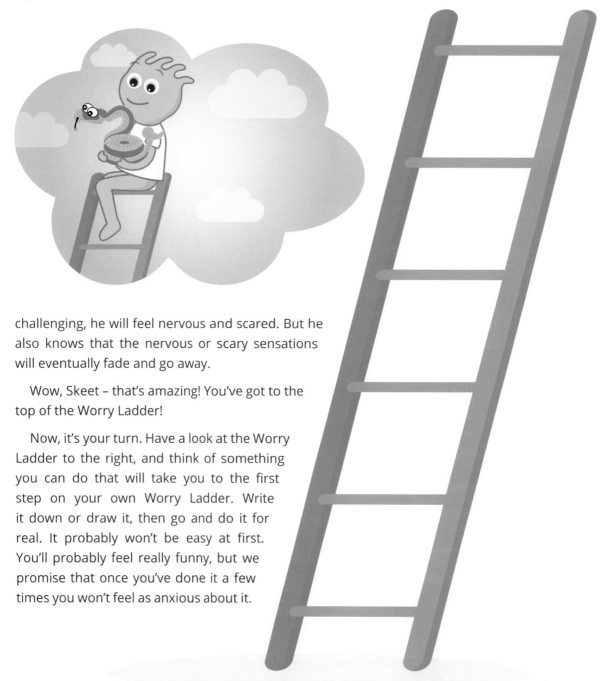

challenging, he will feel nervous and scared. But he also knows that the nervous or scary sensations will eventually fade and go away.

Wow, Skeet – that's amazing! You've got to the top of the Worry Ladder!

Now, it's your turn. Have a look at the Worry Ladder to the right, and think of something you can do that will take you to the first step on your own Worry Ladder. Write it down or draw it, then go and do it for real. It probably won't be easy at first. You'll probably feel really funny, but we promise that once you've done it a few times you won't feel as anxious about it.

Try and set yourself some little targets first and then make them bigger and bigger. For example, if you're nervous about putting your hand up in class, set yourself a target of putting your hand up just once in the first week. Next week, you can do it twice. And the week after that, you can do it more and more …

Skeet spent quite a while looking at the snake pictures, and he stroked the snake several times before deciding he'd like to hold it. Once you've done it, don't forget to celebrate your big achievement. And then you can think about the next step, and the next, and the next, until you've reached the top of the ladder!!

How did you get on? Did you take the first step?

How did you feel? Proud? Surprised? Brave? Hopeful?

Whatever you felt, you certainly deserve a round of applause for making the effort and being so brave!

Talk to the hand!

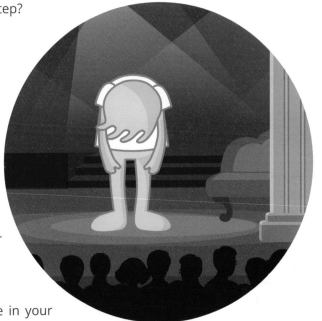

As we know, telling your worries to 'go away' doesn't always work. So let's accept that they are there, but try to ignore them – a bit like an annoying wasp in a room!

So here goes ...

Find a comfortable place to be – maybe in your bedroom, where you are surrounded by your toys, books and pictures. Close your eyes for a moment, and think about your worry ...

When you've done that, open your eyes, have a look at your favourite toy or picture or gadget and talk about what it is, what it looks like, why you like it – everything!!

Then, when you've done that, ask yourself how you felt about doing it? The question is ... did you notice your worry??

If not, well done! That means you ignored it. And if you ignored it once, you can ignore it again and again until it shrinks to nothing. Remember – you can try this in all sorts of places. For example, if you're on a bus and you start to worry about something, just try closing your eyes, thinking about your worry for a moment or two, then opening your eyes and looking at everyone's shoes. See if you can spot all the blue shoes. Or spot the shoes you like best.

This is something you can do in lots of situations. See if you can come up with some ideas of your own. What would you do if you experienced a big worry while you were out shopping? Or at school? The more you try it, the easier it will get.

How to relax

Now, after all that hard work learning about our worries and how we can deal with them, it's time for some

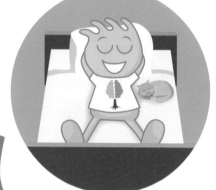

Relaxation

Relaxation is very important for everyone, but it's especially important for people who worry a lot. And so is

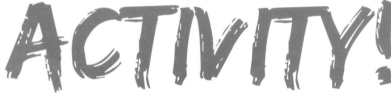

ACTIVITY!

When we worry, our bodies feel tense and nervous. That's because we are on alert for 'danger' – just like those confused cavemen we heard about who were trying to decide whether to fight, run away or freeze. So we need to find things to do things to loosen our bodies and help us feel calm once again.

Skeet likes to relax at home, and he makes time to do things he enjoys that he can concentrate on. This helps him to settle down and forget about Worry for a while.

Skeet does a lot of things that you probably do too, like:

Petting his dog.

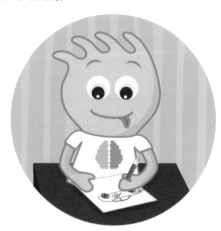

Colouring, drawing and writing.

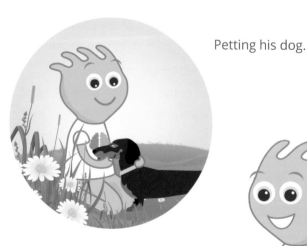

Playing football in the park.

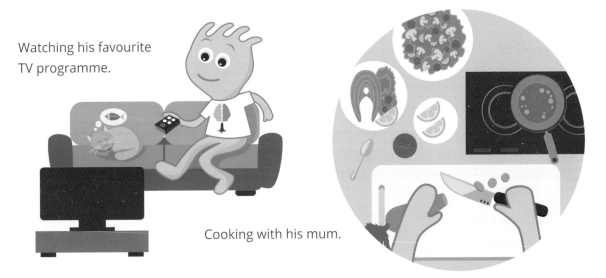

Watching his favourite
TV programme.

Cooking with his mum.

There are loads more ways to relax – and even if you don't think you're relaxing, doing the things you enjoy means that you probably are!

In the box below, draw a picture of yourself doing something that you like. Or draw an activity that makes you feel relaxed.

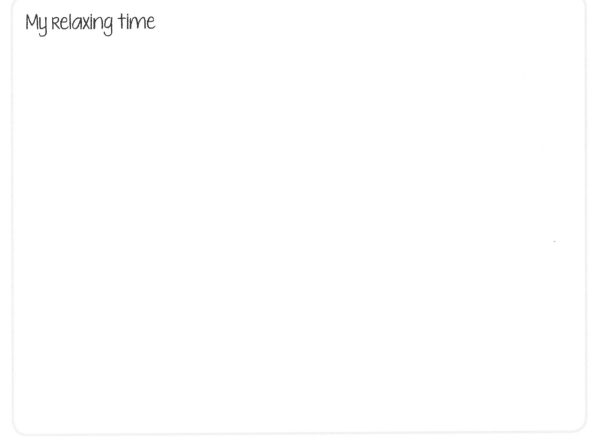

My Relaxing time

Okay, so how did you feel at the end of this? Relaxed?

I hope so!!!

Time to chill!

There are other ways to relax without having to do anything. We'll show you how you can relax the body, and help to release any tense feelings you might have ...

First, lie down or sit in a comfortable position in a quiet room. When you have settled down, tense the muscles in your feet, legs, arms, hands and even your face. If you haven't done this before, imagine you're screwing them up tight. When they all feel 'tight', relax each part of your body, bit by bit.

Start with your feet ...

... then your legs ...

... now let your tummy relax ...

... and your chest ...

... now let your fingers go soft ...

... and let your arms flop by your sides ...

... finally, relax the muscles in your face ...

Open the memory box

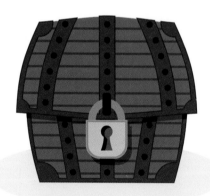

Now, for this exercise we're going to explore some great memories. Think about a time when you were having a lot of fun. Maybe it was on your birthday ... or on your summer holiday. Maybe you were just out and about with your friends. Try to remember as much about it as possible. What could you see? What could you hear? How did you feel? Who else was there?

Okay, now you've got that memory, lock it away in your Memory Box below (write or draw your fun moment in here ...)

Next time you feel a bit worried, go and find your Quiet Place. Next, concentrate on your breathing – breathe in deeply through your nose and out slowly through your mouth. Do this five times, then open your Memory Box and take out your favourite fun memory. Replay it in your mind like a short video. You can pretend you have a remote control and rewind it, or even fast forward to the most fun bit and rewind it again.

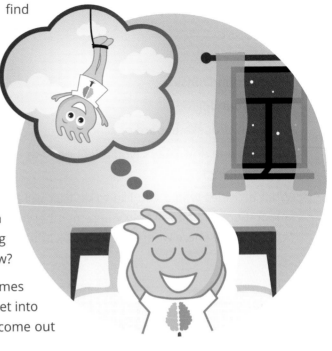

When your 'video' has finished, lie still for a few moments then carry on what you were doing before you started to relax. How do you feel now?

If you do this every day, or even just a few times a week, you'll be amazed how quickly you can get into your 'happy space' and feel brilliant when you come out of it.

Get up and go!

As well as relaxing, you can also beat worry by being active. Lots of people who exercise find that it stops them from feeling stressed and worried, because exercise sends lots of great chemicals from the brain to the body.

The more we exercise, the more our brain sends out these signals to our body that we can be excited and active, rather than stressed and worried – and at the same time we become fitter and stronger too! Skeet's friend Susan sometimes felt tense. So to help, a friend suggested that she did ten 'Star Jumps' whenever she felt that way.

After she did them, she was really out of breath. But the good news was – the tension in her body had disappeared!!

Susan was burning off all the nervous energy that was being made in her body. After the star jumps she felt much better.

You can do star jumps too. You can also:

- Play sport
- Ride your bike
- Run around outside
- Walk your dog
- Play on your skateboard or scooter
- Run up and downstairs (you might need to tell your parents or caregivers so they know what you're doing)

What activities would you like to do that will chase the anxious feelings and worry away? Think about them, or, if it will help you remember make a list and put it in your favourite book, on your wall, or somewhere where you can look at it when you want to.

Chapter 12

How to Beat OCD

For parents and caregivers: This section deals with OCD in children, and teaches both you and your child ways to deal with the problem. In Part I, Chapter 8 we discussed OCD in detail, so before you start this part of the recovery approach with your child, you might find it helpful to re-read that chapter.

To recap, OCD is an obsessional problem that can be about anything, causing us to feel anxious, depressed, ashamed and guilty. In brief, OCD is when people have intrusions that are very upsetting, which they interpret as being very threatening, so they feel worried, anxious and fearful, and naturally want to minimise or reduce the threat, or stop themselves having these intrusions in the first place.

OCD shares a lot of similarities with Worry but with OCD, importance is attached to thought; the child feels responsible for preventing harm in some way and may feel very strongly that they must get rid of these feelings or the worrying thoughts or images, so they respond to the fear in a ritualised and compulsive way. The child with OCD might have counting rituals, checking rituals, repetitive behaviours, mental compulsions (for example, 'trying to solve the problem' in their head, or 'ruminating' – repeatedly going over the same worry). They may seek reassurance by asking the same things over and over, and try to avoid things that they think might make the intrusions come true, or to prevent themselves having more worrying thoughts and feelings. We have referred to these responses generally as 'safety behaviours' because they are actions that people with anxiety and obsessional problems, including OCD, carry out to feel safe from the feared outcome of their worries. They might work for a while but they will not make the worries go away in the long term.

The child with OCD will certainly benefit from the last few chapters about Worry, so please take the time to go over them with your child before working on this one.

The biggest piece of advice to parents and caregivers with a child who has OCD is to try to intervene in their compulsions or rituals. It is hard for children to stop rituals, compulsions and safety behaviours themselves, because they find it difficult to understand why the things that they believe are keeping them 'safe', stopping harm from occurring or preventing them from feeling anxious, should have to go.

When you intervene in a ritual or compulsion, your child might scream, cry, or throw a tantrum. We understand that it is very hard to see your child in a state of distress, but please be assured that you are doing the right thing by intervening in a ritual or compulsion. This kind of reaction is perfectly normal; even adults with OCD experience high levels of stress if their safety behaviours are removed. If you don't intervene the ritual may continue, and become more complicated, and the OCD may start interfering in their lives in new ways.

Here are just a few of the ways you can stop the ritual or compulsive behaviour:

- Interrupt routines or counting rituals (e.g. not allowing the light to be switched on and off multiple times)
- Interrupt mental counting when you can see it happening
- Limit showering to five minutes or handwashing to thirty seconds where appropriate (i.e. clearly dirty hands or after using the toilet) and not allowing extra showers etc.
- Tidy rooms or put things away that you know they don't want you to touch
- Don't give in to unreasonable requests for checking etc.
- Change the order of things that have been placed in a particular way
- Stop avoiding places as requested by your child

These are only a handful of suggestions for intervening, and you might come up with your own unique ideas, depending on your child's compulsion and safety behaviour. It is very useful to explain to children that what you're doing together is a type of experiment on their 'unhelpful habits', and that while they may feel bad while the experiment is happening, the more they take part in the experiments, the quicker the unpleasant feelings will go away. To help with this, you could encourage your child to carry out some 'helpful distractions' (such as exercise, reading, watching TV or socialising with friends) instead of carrying out their compulsions. Don't worry. We're not replacing one form of avoidance with another. You are helping your child do something constructive while they wait for the uncomfortable feelings to pass.

In addition, we'd also like to repeat the advice NOT to reassure your child that we made at the beginning of the book. Reassurance very often reinforces anxiety and OCD, and 'enough reassurance' is never enough. It is hard, especially around children, not to comfort sufferers by reassurance, but it is the right way.

For example, I had a young client, David, who used to ask his mother to check his hands were clean after washing them. His obsession was about dirt and spreading dirt around his room and his toys, and no amount of reassurance from his mum was enough. So whenever he asked her to check his hands she said: 'I'm not going to answer that as it is an unhelpful question like we discussed.'

At first, David was upset and yelled at his mum but eventually he stopped and accepted that she was not going to offer the reassurance he wanted.

Around the same time, David's mum stopped buying soap or keeping anti-bacterial wipes around for the toilet, as she noticed both items being used too much.

Instead, she encouraged David to play with his toys and touch things in his room straight after coming inside from school. Eventually, David stopped worrying so much as he wanted to play computer games and his reassurance-seeking behaviour died down.

Now back to the kids:
What is OCD?

OCD is a funny term. We hear it a lot these days. If you switch a light on and off a few times, or you keep checking in a cupboard, or you don't like getting your hands dirty while you're playing outside, people might say, 'Oh, you're a bit OCD!'

Checking things sometimes, and trying to keep clean isn't OCD. It's just normal stuff. Real OCD interferes in your life by making you worried that something bad or harmful will happen if you don't keep clean, or you don't check the lights are off, or carry out another OCD ritual.

Did you know, we have thousands and thousands of thoughts every day? You're probably not even aware of most of them. Sometimes we have really odd thoughts, or get weird images in our head. Sometimes we have doubts about things, or we get the urge to do things.

The strange thoughts, images, urges and doubts are a bit like worries (in fact, they often ARE worries). Most of the time, they come into our heads and go out again. These can be things like worrying that your parents or caregivers will get ill, or thinking that you've caused an accident. You might even worry that you want to randomly shout out swear words in a quiet library or at the cinema!

But sometimes – like Worries – they get stuck. And when this happens, the strange thoughts, images, urges and doubts have nowhere to escape to. So instead they just keep going round and round and round in your head.

It's a bit like hearing your favourite song, then listening to it going round your brain for days afterwards. That's a nice feeling. But imagine it is a song you really HATE!

Do you know this feeling? If you do, you'll know that you'd do ANYTHING to get the terrible song out of your head.

You might put your fingers in your ears.

Or you might try to think of something else.

Or you might even say some magic words that will make it disappear!

You might be lucky and make it disappear. But the problem with trying very hard to get rid of it is that the terrible song usually comes back!

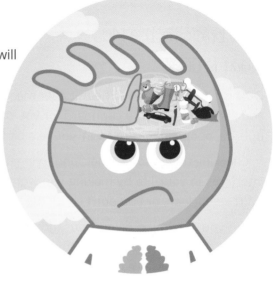

It's the same with strange thoughts, images, urges and doubts. They keep going around in your head. So you try to 'push' them away by doing different things. But it's really hard to make them go away and stay away. Often they just come back, even bigger than before.

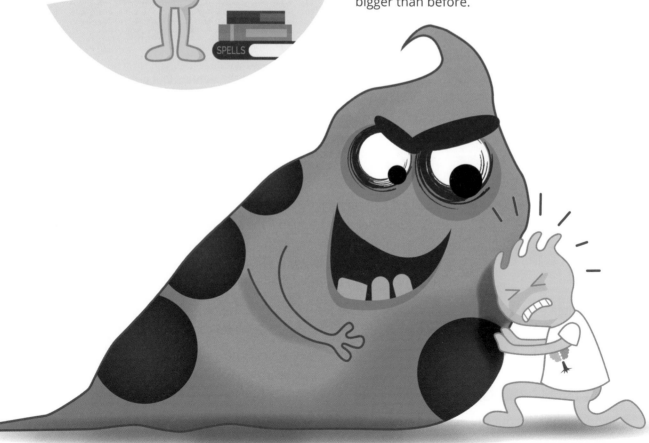

Trying to stop it all

If you're worried about something bad happening, you might also do something to try to stop it. If Skeet's friend Jayne worries about her dad driving to work every day, and has images of him being in a car crash, she might count to 20 every morning and night because she believes this will stop her dad's car from crashing.

Every day that Jayne's dad comes home safely, it makes Jayne feel like the 'magic' is working. So she keeps doing it. But the bad feeling is strong, and it will probably come back soon, worse than ever!

So what IS OCD?

The term 'OCD' is made up of three big words. The first is **OBSESSIVE**. Those are the strange thoughts, images, urges, and doubts that are going round in your head and body.

The next word is **COMPULSIVE**. This is the thing (or things) you do to get rid of the troubling thoughts and uncomfortable feelings, and to stop the bad thing from happening that you worry about. This is how you make yourself and others feel 'safe'.

The last word is **DISORDER**. This is something that is a problem because it stops people from living their lives in the way they want.

No wonder people with OCD feel so anxious. And when we feel anxious we try to get rid of these strange thoughts, images, urges and doubts. That is why we carry out compulsions, or rituals, like counting to 20, or turning light switches on and off.

So together that makes Obsessive-Compulsive Disorder – OCD! This describes the feeling of a funny, silly or upsetting thought, image, urge or doubt that gets stuck in your mind. And that's what makes us feel so anxious. OCD also describes the things you do to try to get rid of the uncomfortable thoughts or feelings, or to stop the thing you worry about from happening.

OCD can be scary. The strange thoughts, images, urges, and doubts that you've had suddenly get serious, and worse still, they get stuck in your head. It makes you feel strange, and you think you need to do something to stop bad things happening, or to 'unstick' your thought and get rid of it, so that you can get rid of all the unpleasant feelings that come with them.

The good news is that your thoughts aren't stuck forever – you can deal with them and feel better!!

There are two boxes below. In the left-hand box, write down or draw any strange or funny thoughts you've had which you think have become stuck. In the right-hand box, write down or draw the ways you've tried to get rid of them or stop bad things from happening.

My funny thoughts and images, and what I worry might happen ...

How I've tried to get rid of them!

As we've said, trying to get rid of the funny thoughts or to stop things from happening doesn't really work. In fact, it sometimes makes them more scary. Let's see what happened to Skeet ...

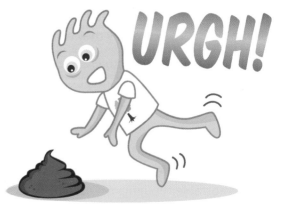

One day, when he was playing football in the field, Skeet tripped and put his hand into some dog poo. UGHHH!! Disgusting!!

Everyone laughed at him, and he felt very dirty and embarrassed (even though it wasn't his fault).

When he got home, his mum said that he needed to be more careful, because he could get germs from dog poo. She said that if he washed his hands, he would be alright. So he washed his hands, then he felt okay again.

After that, Skeet began to think a lot about germs. 'You can pass germs to other people,' he thought, 'and make them ill. You might even make them die ...' Skeet worried a lot about this thought. He worried about passing on germs to his little sister and his grandma, and making them ill. So he started to wash his hands more often, and for longer and longer. And when he washed them, he felt much better.

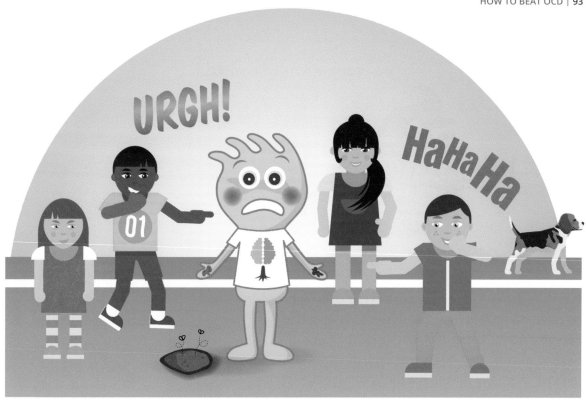

Soon, Skeet came to believe that whatever worry he had would go away if he washed his hands, even though these worries were nothing to do with being dirty. And he washed, and washed, and washed ... until ...

His hands were so red and sore, he had to go to the doctor to get some special cream, and he explained to the doctor why he had to wash his hands so much. The doctor said he didn't have to wash so much, but Skeet didn't believe him because washing his hands made him feel better.

And all of this happened just because a thought about germs got stuck in Skeet's mind. Skeet thought it would be his fault if someone he knew caught germs and got ill.

Do you think it would be his fault?

Or can anyone catch germs anywhere?

Because washing his hands helped Skeet stop worrying about germs, he thought that washing his hands would help him deal with all his worries. So how does washing hands help a worry that doesn't involve dirt? The answer is, it doesn't!

And if you think that anyone can catch germs anywhere, you're right! Everyone picks up and passes on germs. It's part of being human. Skeet had a silly thought about germs that he took **too seriously**. That's what happens with OCD – it wants you to take it seriously, because it wants to boss you about and tell you what to do.

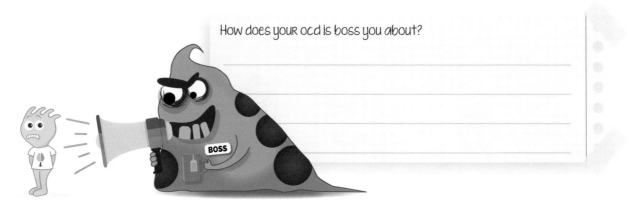

How does your ocd is boss you about?

Bossy OCD!

But if we let OCD become the boss, it will keep bossing us around and making us do things to keep it happy. People with OCD can feel exhausted because they have to work so hard to try and keep the unpleasant feelings quiet and to stop the funny thoughts and images.

Do you remember Skeet's friend Jayne?

Jayne is very close to her granny, and loves her very much. When Jayne's granny became ill, Jayne started to worry that she might die. The upsetting images just popped into her head (like a little film), but these are actually very normal thoughts because we worry about the people we love.

Jayne's granny went into hospital and was well looked after by the doctors and nurses. Jayne kept thinking that her gran would die because she had the image in her head, and she felt very bad for having that thought. So to make it go away, she did two things. First, she tried to undo the bad image. Lots of people who have OCD try to do this. It means she tried to replace the 'scary' image of her gran dying with a 'good' one of her at home, talking to Jayne about what she'd been doing at school.

The second thing Jayne did was to count to 20.

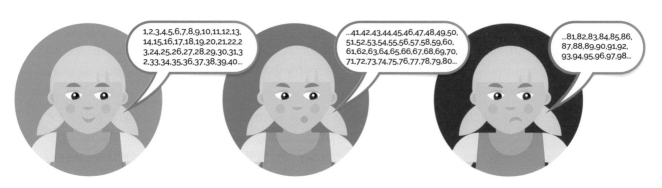

But the thought didn't go away. So she counted to 40 …

But the thought still didn't go away. So she counted to 80 …

And even then, the thought didn't go away! So she counted to 100.

… but when she got to 98, Jayne's mum shouted, 'Jayne! It's time for tea!' And her counting had to stop right there!

Because Jayne didn't manage to count to 100, she had to start all over again. This made her late for her ballet lesson, and her teacher was cross. It wasn't Jayne's fault – it was her OCD, bossing her around!

In the end, Jayne's granny got better and came out of hospital. But Jayne kept thinking about her dying, and feeling bad that she had that image. And she kept counting and counting, hoping that it would keep her granny safe. She started to count lamp posts on her way to school, and would get very upset if her mum drove past each lamp post too quickly for Jayne to count it properly.

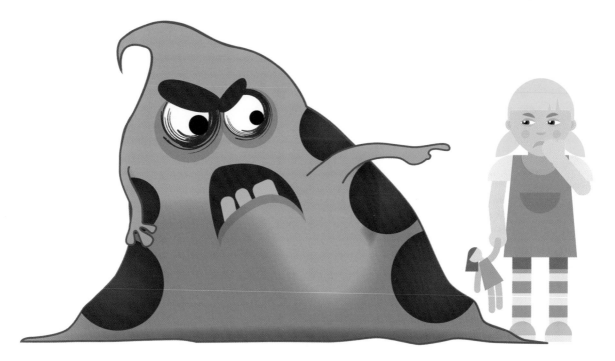

And guess what? Jayne stopped doing all the things she liked doing because she spent so much of her time counting. Her granny got better because she was given medicine, not because Jayne was counting! So really, the whole thing was just a big waste of time. But that's OCD being sneaky because it made her think that it made her grandmother better! But we know it wasn't OCD. It was the helpful doctors and nurses and the medicines they gave her.

The Worry Wheel

Skeet and Jayne both have what we call a Worry Wheel. This is a bit like one of those fireworks that whirl round, faster and faster, once it is lit.

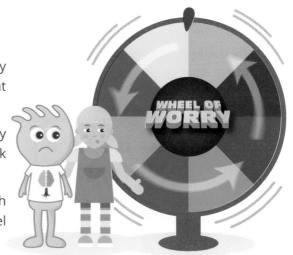

At the top of the wheel is Skeet and Jayne's funny thought. This is like the match that lights the firework and starts it spinning.

This thought makes them both anxious, which drives the wheel even faster and makes them feel shaky, or sick, or sweaty, or frightened.

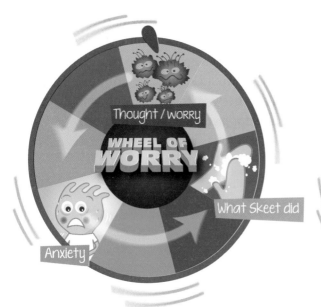

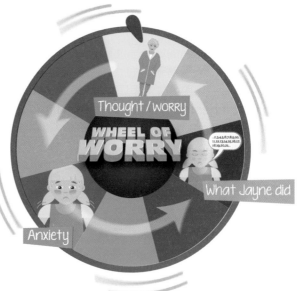

Jayne and Skeet try to do things to slow the wheel down.

But because they're taking their funny thoughts seriously, the wheel doesn't slow down. In fact, it spins faster and faster!

Jayne wants to prevent her gran from dying. Skeet wants to stop himself from feeling dirty. And they're both trying hard to make their strange thoughts, images, urges and doubts go away, but it's not really working.

So what can we do to stop your OCD and make sure it's not bullying you?

Well, the first and most important thing is to tell mum and dad (or an adult you trust) that you're having strange thoughts, images, urges and doubts. Tell them that you're having to do some strange things (like counting, or repeating words in your head) to get rid of them or stop something bad from happening, but it isn't working. Asking someone to help you is not embarrassing or silly. We understand how strange and scary it feels to have strange thoughts, images, urges and doubts in your head, but if you keep them locked away there, they will only get worse. If OCD was a real person, and he was bullying you, you'd tell someone straight away, wouldn't you?

So think of OCD as a big bully. The more attention you give your bully, the more he's going to want to make your life a misery ...

It's time to tell someone about him!!

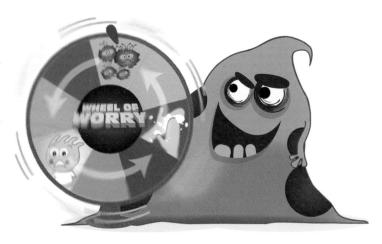

Mum and dad might have noticed you counting, or washing your hands, or blinking, or checking locks and doors, or doing whatever you do to keep your OCD quiet. So now is the time to try some experiments with them. We're going to play scientists again!

Before we become scientists, take a moment to think about your own worry wheel. You can fill in the blank worry wheel below with your worrying thoughts, how you felt and what you did because you had the worrying thought.

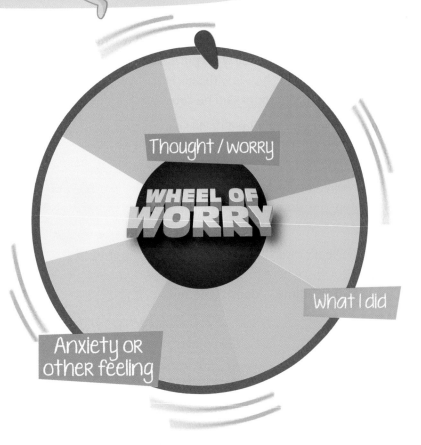

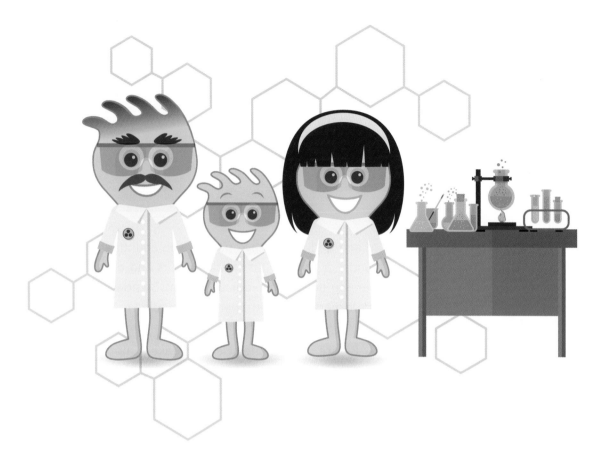

How to experiment

When Skeet told his parents about dog poo and germs, and washing his hands, they thought the best idea was for Skeet to get his hands dirty on purpose. This was hard for Skeet at first, but he went into the garden and rubbed his hands with soil. He felt very funny, but he had the soil on his hands for five minutes before his parents said he could wash it off.

The next day, Skeet's parents asked him if he'd like to try getting his hands dirty AND not washing them! This was hard for Skeet at first, because he was still worrying about passing on germs. Not washing his hands would feel really uncomfortable, and he knew it would be hard to stop the urge to wash his hands straightaway.

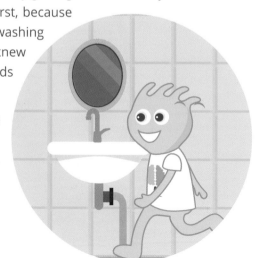

'We understand,' said Skeet's mum and dad, 'and we know it will be difficult. But we're here to support you, and if you don't get it right first time, it doesn't matter. As long as you try ...'

So he tried ...

And he tried ...

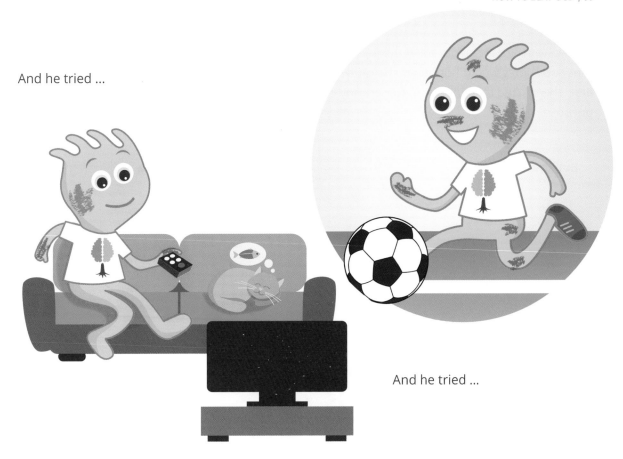

And he tried ...

Skeet really didn't like eating dinner with dirty hands, but he was so interested in his favourite TV programme that he forgot all about his hands. He definitely wasn't sure about going to bed with dirty hands, but he did it anyway. And when he woke up, he realised he was still alright. Nothing bad had happened.

So Skeet realised that not washing his hands didn't mean he would pass on germs. He still washed them after using the toilet, or when there was dirt on them (after helping his dad in the garden), and sometimes before dinner (when he remembered!) but he stopped washing them all the time. Which means he now has more time for all the things he likes doing. And most importantly, he has shut up his OCD.

When Jayne told her mum about counting lamp posts, she said that if she saw Jayne counting, she would interrupt her. This sounds a bit mean, but it isn't. So Jayne and her mum went out on a drive. Whenever they did this in the past, they had to stop at every lamp post because Jayne wanted to count it.

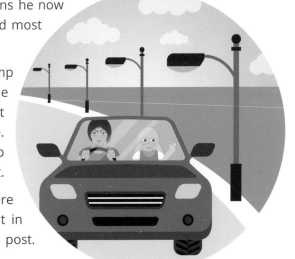

This made Jayne's mum cross, because they were always late for everything! So when they went out in the car again, Jayne's mum didn't stop at the lamp post. Instead, she drove past.

This was hard for Jayne, and it upset her. She still worried that bad things would happen if she didn't count. And at first, she started thinking about her granny getting ill on purpose.

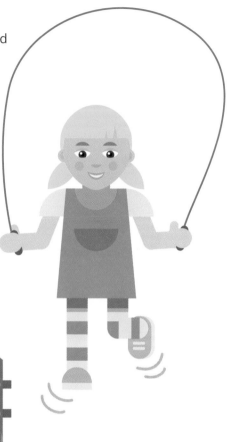

But she tried ...

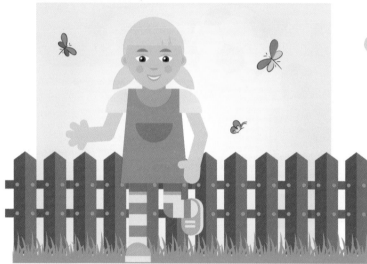

And she tried ...

And finally, she realised that counting didn't mean bad things (or even good things) would happen! And now she is never late and has much more time to do the things she enjoys. She doesn't let her OCD boss her around any more, and these days the things she likes counting best are the sweets that her granny gives her when she goes to visit!

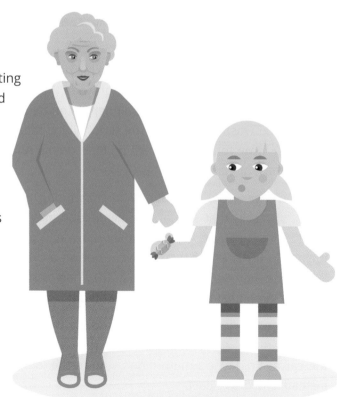

You are the scientist!

Okay, now it's your turn to be the scientist. With your mum or dad (or both) you're going to see what happens to your OCD when you experiment on it. Just remember, when we do these experiments, we are deliberately trying to make ourselves feel uncomfortable. That's the best way to prove that these feelings won't last forever. We can make them disappear quickly.

What are you going to have to do?

Well, if you're worried about dirt, you can try putting your hands in dirty places. Or if you're worried about keeping things in the right order all the time, you'll have to try not lining things up right. Or, if keeping lots of things helps make you feel better, you're going to have to throw some things away on purpose.

Your experiment is to **do the opposite** of what your OCD is telling you! When Skeet was worried about passing on germs, he experimented with not washing his hands. When Jayne kept counting lamp posts, she experimented with not counting them. When they did the opposite of what their OCD wanted them to do, they saw that bad things didn't happen just because they had stopped doing what their OCD told them to do.

In the box below, write down what you normally do to stop your worries, then write down the experiment you're going to use to interrupt them.

When I have an OCD worry, these are the things I do to try and get rid of it, to stop the bad thing from happening, or to try and stop feeling uncomfortable …

_____

_____

_____

_____

what my experiment is …

_____

_____

How ocd will try and get in the way?

_____

_____

_____

_____

What do I need to do to make sure the ocd doesn't stop me from trying this experiment?

_____

_____

_____

What happened when I tried my experiment?

_____

_____

_____

What is my next experiment?

_____

When you do your experiments you have to be a scientist ... and a knight! In other words, you need to be brave. That's not always easy, but if you keep practising ...

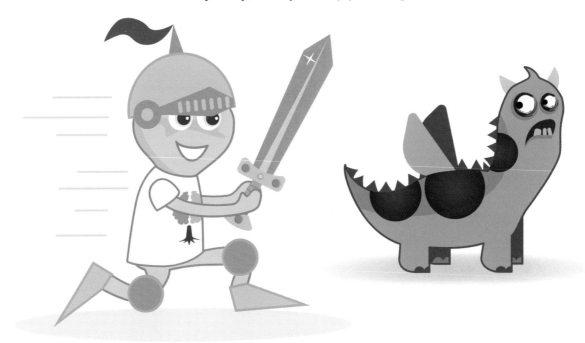

You will become brave and strong, and you will be able to get on top of your OCD easily!

Have you tried your experiment yet? If so, give yourself a BIG round of applause!

Now, let's think about what happened when you did your experiment ...

How did you feel when you were doing it?

How did you feel an hour later?

How did you feel that night?

Do you think you could do it again?

You probably felt really uncomfortable for a while ... but did you stop noticing that feeling after a bit?

Scientists often try the same experiment again to try and see if there are any differences. So, why not give it another go? Then ask yourself the same questions.

Don't forget, every time you try the experiment, it will get easier. The more you do it, the more comfortable you'll feel.

Chapter 13

Life Beyond Worry and OCD

Feeling great again

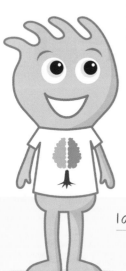

Do you remember the questions we asked you about yourself? Well, you are still that person, but you can add that you are very brave for tackling your worries so successfully!

You are amazing, and ...

You know how to tackle that big bully, your OCD. What a hero!

Below, think about what you were most proud of when you were tackling your worries? What did you find hard? What did you find easy? What worked best for you?

I am proud of ...

_____

_____

_____

Next, you might find it helpful to write down all the good things about yourself, and all the good things other people say about you. This is really important, because when a bully – like OCD – picks on you, it makes you feel bad about yourself, and it makes you feel weak and helpless. But now you know that you're brave and courageous, not weak and helpless!

The good stuff about me ...

_____

_____

_____

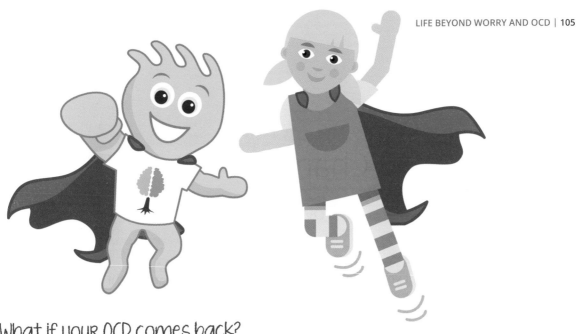

What if your OCD comes back?

Now you've faced down the twin bullies of Worry and OCD. Great, you can do all the things you enjoy doing again. But, how can you guarantee that your worries and your OCD won't come back?

The answer is – you can't!

There are no guarantees in life. Things happen that you can't control. But you CAN train your Worry or OCD to make sure they stay as far away from you as possible.

We've seen how you can make Worry shrink away, and how you can stop OCD bullying you. So if you ever feel that they're hanging around, follow the exercises and do the experiments that helped you this time. And if you feel Worry and OCD coming back, tell someone!

Bullies only like it when someone is frightened of them. If they're being ignored, or challenged, they tend to go away. So remember to be brave, just like Skeet and Jayne were.

You might also find it helpful to write down some advice (in the box below) that you would give to someone else with worries …

My advice is …

_____

_____

_____

_____

Once Worry and OCD have shrunk, remember your knight's training. Keep exercising, sleeping well and eating healthy food. If you build a healthy body, you will develop a healthy mind, and this will protect you from Worry and OCD.

Chapter 14

The Power of Sleep

Sleeping is very important. If you have a good night's sleep, you feel great. But if you have a bad night's sleep, you feel a bit like a tired, angry monster!

Because you're still young, you need lots of sleep. It's good for your body and your mind, especially if you're dealing with worry and OCD. If you don't get enough sleep, it can make it harder to concentrate at school. Not getting enough sleep can make you feel sad and depressed too.

If you are already dealing with feelings of anxiety, you need to be extra careful to get enough sleep, because the more tired you are, the more anxious you'll feel.

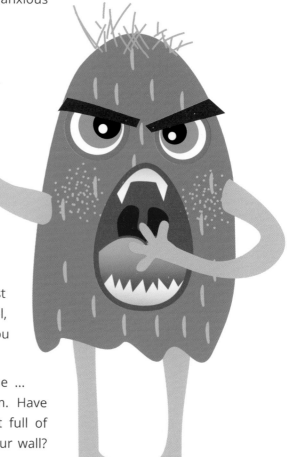

Don't worry ... In this chapter we'll tell you what you can do to make going to bed a really nice part of your day.

Just how much sleep do you need?

Probably more than you think! Up to the age of nine, you still need between 10 and 11 hours' sleep a night! Even 16-year-olds are recommended to get their nine hours of sleep a night!

If you find it hard to get to sleep, we can help. Just like getting up in the morning and being at school, you'll find that getting to sleep is much easier if you have a good routine.

We can help you make a great bedtime routine ... But first, let's have a think about your bedroom. Have a think about your room. What colour is it? Is it full of toys and teddies? Have you got any posters on your wall? Can you see your bed, or is it covered in stuff?

Keep it tidy!

We know that people with anxiety find it easier to sleep in a tidy, organised room. (Your mum or dad will like this bit!) If there are too many exciting things happening in your room – too many posters or toys to catch your attention, it will make it more difficult to get to sleep. Try to keep your room tidy so that there is nothing to distract you when you go to bed.

Try not to have too much light in your room. As it gets darker, our bodies start to get ready for sleep. So if your room is too light, it will make it much harder to get to sleep. You can have a little night light if you like.

Some people like to listen to calming sounds when they go to bed. Ask your mum or dad about playing some relaxing sounds like waves on a beach, or some classical music – which many people find very relaxing.

Eat right

What we eat is really important. But when we eat is important too. So here are some tips for you:

- At your last meal of the day as early as you can.
- Cut down on sugary, fizzy drinks. Lots of them contain caffeine which keeps people awake!
- Don't have too many sugary snacks – especially later in the day. You don't want all that sugar to leave you buzzing with energy just before bedtime!
- If you like a night-time drink before bed, try a nice mug of warm milk, and ask mum or dad if they can sprinkle a bit of nutmeg on top. Nutmeg is a bit of a wonder spice which aids relaxation.

Exercise and sleep

Remember all those busy days when mum or dad says, 'You'll sleep well tonight!' – well it's true. Children who get plenty of exercise in the day sleep better at night. Even better, exercise beats stress – so it's a great way to tackle anxiety.

Here are some things you can do after school to get a little extra exercise:

- Try an after-school sports club.
- Have a little walk, a bike ride or a kick around before dinner.
- Get some friends over and get them out in the back garden to burn off some energy.
- Take a trip to the park or the playground.
- Take a dance class, or try a martial art.

Screen time

A bit of TV every day is fine. Just not too much. And not straight before bed.

Do you like computer games? You can still play computer games, but not for an hour or so before bed. We know that games can make you tense, anxious and excitable – three things we don't want you to be right before you try to sleep.

You'll need to turn your phone and tablet off an hour before bed too, I'm afraid. The screens are just too bright – and what your body really needs before sleep is darkness.

Your perfect bedtime

Knowing that you have a set bedtime routine can really help reassure you. Better yet, having an hour filled with relaxing bathtime, stories, and talking with you can become a really nice part of your day.

Here are some good ideas that people use to help them sleep. Talk about these ideas with your mum and dad and see if you can create your perfect bedtime routine ...

Seven tips for a stress-free bedtime routine:

1) No more checking phones or tablets, no computer games, no TV. All of these things excite your brain, and make it much harder to relax and get sleepy.

2) The temperature of your body drops just before you fall asleep. So if you have 15 or 20 minutes in a nice warm bath, your body temperature will rise and then start to dip when you get out, just ready for bed.

3) Remember when we talked about relaxation? Take another look at page 82 if you need a reminder. It's a very good way to deal with your anxiety in a positive way. It can really help you calm down before bedtime. Ask Mum and Dad if they can find out more for you, or get a book from the library.

4) To keep bedtime as stress-free as possible, don't make too many decisions. Make sure you know what toy you're going to take to bed, what book you're going to read and which pyjamas you're going to wear. Keep it simple.

5) Enjoy reading with Mum or Dad for 10–15 minutes. Get cosy, snuggle up, and enjoy the story.

6) After your story, it's okay to have a few minutes talking-time with Mum or Dad. This can be a really nice chance to talk over some of the things that have happened in your day.

7) Time for hugs and goodnight kisses.

Try it. I think that you'll enjoy your new routine. It might take a few days to get used to it, but stick with it.

Emergency sleep tips!

You've got a great new sleep routine going, but suppose it doesn't work one night? What then?

Don't worry, your sleep routine isn't 'broken'. We all have nights when we just can't drop off to sleep. Maybe you've just got too many thoughts buzzing round your brain.

So what do you do?

It's a good idea to talk to mum or dad about what you can do if you wake up in the night. They might have some good ideas for you. Here are a few to get you started …

The worst thing you can do when you can't sleep is to lie there worrying about the fact you're not asleep. Go and talk to Mum or Dad if they're still awake. Or, if you're worried about something, write it down! It's surprising how much better it can feel when you've put your worries on paper. It's like taking them out of your mind and storing them somewhere else so you can sleep.

It can help your mind relax if you stay out of bed for a little while – pop your dressing gown on so you don't get cold and read a book for 10 or 15 minutes. Choose a comfy chair and head back to bed when you've finished. This is a good way to stop your brain worrying and let it relax, before heading back to bed.

Chapter 15

Be Brilliant!

How did you feel when you beat your worry and OCD?

In the box below, write about, or draw a picture about how you felt when you started to beat your worries and OCD. Describe how it felt to feel brilliant.

I started to beat my worries and OCD and I felt ...

_____

_____

_____

_____

_____

_____

_____

Can you stop your worries coming back?

You will always have some worries in your life. We all do. But that's okay. Because now you know how to deal with them.

So if you ever feel a bit down in the dumps, or worried, try to remember how it felt when you beat your worry or OCD, and when you drew this picture to show how it felt. Then - plan something that you'll really enjoy doing!

My toolbox

Remember – you now have a big box of tools that you can use to send away Worry and OCD.

You don't have to use them all at once – just remember to pick the ones you find are the most useful. Why don't you write these down below? They might include:

- Telling our family that we have funny thoughts, images, doubts or feelings.
- Doing the experiments to see what actually happens.
- Having our family help us with the experiments.
- Finding out that it's okay to feel uncomfortable.
- Thinking good things about ourselves, and hearing the nice things other people say about us.
- Doing things that help us relax.
- Taking care not to fall into thinking traps.
- Finding new ways to think about our worries – creating a new story for ourselves.
- Ignoring worry.
- Having a good night's sleep.

My most useful tools to send away Worry and OCD are:

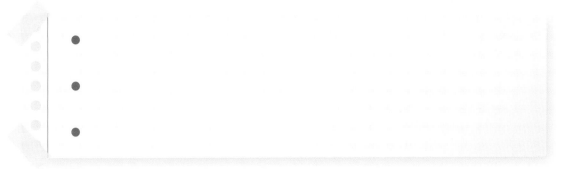

Things I found helpful during my quest to beat my worry and OCD include:

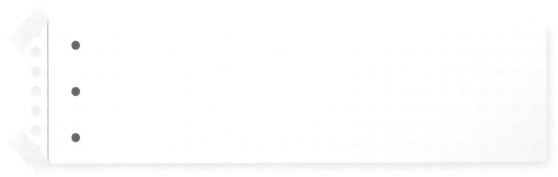

What I will do if I notice my worries or OCD coming back?

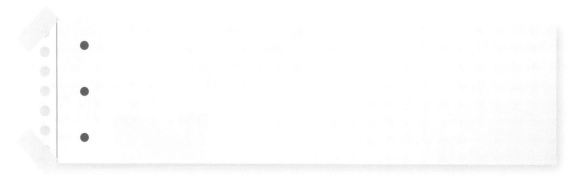

If you feel Worry and OCD coming back, try not to worry. Treat it just like any other illness. If you get a cold, you know you're going to feel a bit rubbish for a few days, so you keep warm, have plenty of hot drinks, stay in bed, and get a good night's sleep. You rest, you take it easy, and you start to feel a bit better. And just like a cold, if you prepare for OCD and Worry, you'll have all the tools you need to send them packing.

One final thing - you might find it helpful to draw a picture of yourself, or take a selfie, showing how you want to look when you are free of Worry and OCD in the box below. You could also draw the medal you'd like to award yourself for being so brave. When you've done it, take a photo of it and stick it on your wall.

Be proud. You have done something amazing. You have beaten your bullies and now you're ready for anything!!

This is me - free of Worry and / or OCD!

Managing Anxiety in Teenagers

Chapter 16

Getting to Grips with Anxiety

 Lauren: Hi, and welcome to the teenagers' section. In the next few chapters I'll help you understand and get to grips with anxiety, worry, and OCD. Together, we'll come up with a plan to beat the worries, obsessions, and habits that are causing you problems.

Before we really get down to business, I'd like you to read Adam's story, in Part I, Chapter 1 of this book. Adam had OCD – a type of anxiety problem which involves worry. Of course, you can also have anxiety and worry without having OCD, so Adam's story is just as relevant for people without OCD who have excessive worry and anxiety.

Come back when you've read it and we'll concentrate on you...

Now, I know you are having some difficulties right now, but don't let that cloud your judgement. I'm sure there are people in your life who think you're amazing. And, I have to say, you get a lot of respect from me because you've decided to do something about the difficulties you're having – and that takes a lot of courage.

WORRIES AND ANXIETIES

What do we mean when we talk about worry and anxiety? The words are often swapped for each other, which is fine, but technically speaking WORRIES are the thoughts that you have, and ANXIETY is the emotion and physical sensations you experience as a result of those worries.

When we use the term 'thoughts' in relation to worry, these include images or pictures in our head, as well as doubts. In OCD we also include urges and sensations in this category. I know this might seem confusing now, but stay with me and hopefully it'll all make sense.

For example, Jen couldn't stop thinking about what other people might be thinking of her. Her WORRY was:

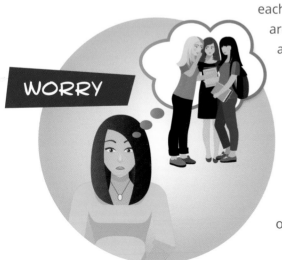

that they were thinking negative things about her. When she thought about it, she felt sick, a bit panicky, self-conscious, fearful and shaky. This is ANXIETY.

If you have worries and anxieties, and you think you have OCD too, this chapter, and the ones after it, will be really useful to you.

Knowing that other people understand some of what you're feeling and experiencing can be a comfort. From reading Adam's story, you'll know that:

• **You're not alone.** Lots of people suffer from anxiety and worry problems in one way or another.

• Our thoughts, sensations, feelings and emotions work to create anxiety and worry – but we can 're-set' them so we **tell ourselves a different story** about what we're thinking, feeling and experiencing. This can break the vicious cycle of anxiety and worry that you feel trapped in.

LET'S BEGIN ...

You're reading this book because you have an anxiety or worry problem which is affecting your life. It might be that your anxiety or worry problem is causing difficulties for you:

• At school

• At home

• At work or on your job training

• With your family

• With friends

• When you're alone

Anxiety and worry can affect you in so many different ways. It may stop you from doing things you used to enjoy, or going places you used to like, or trying new things. It might make you quiet and shy. It might force you to do things (like washing your hands, or checking doors, repeating actions or avoiding people and places) that take up all your valuable time. It can leave you feeling worried, confused, upset, hurt, guilty, nervous and frightened.

But guess what? Anxiety is actually a **completely normal feeling**.

When you're feeling upset and frightened and worried, it isn't easy to accept that anxiety is normal, because it feels like the worst thing in the world.

But everyone experiences anxiety. It's part of who we are. Anyone who says, 'I never, ever worry about anything, ever,' isn't being honest. They say it because they **do worry** about something, and just don't like to show it, or don't consider it a problem for themselves.

When I say that anxiety is 'normal', what I mean is that a **certain level of anxiety** is normal. Before an exam, or on a first date, or making a presentation in class, or before a sports event – all these things come with a bit of anxiety. Most people tend to worry about them beforehand, then go and do the thing they were worried about anyway. Afterwards, they usually find that it wasn't really worth worrying about anyway!

LISTENING TO WORRY

However, not all of us react like this. Some of us listen very hard to our worries:

'You'll never pass the exam,' Worry says, *'so what's the point in even trying?'*

'That girl / boy you're going out on a date with – they're going to make fun of the clothes you're wearing. So it's better not to go at all...'

'That presentation you're making in class – forget it! It's all going to go wrong and everyone will think you're an idiot...'

'No one liked or commented on that Facebook / Twitter / Instagram post you made – everyone must think it's stupid.'

So you see how nasty anxiety and worry can be if you give in to them?

FIGHT, FLIGHT OR FREEZE

Back in prehistoric times, anxiety was very useful when primitive man was faced with a threat. If you saw a sabre-toothed tiger prowling outside your cave, you had three choices:

• Stand up and fight it, in the hope you might win and then have it for dinner.

• Freeze on the spot in the hope it didn't see you, or thought you were dead.

• Run away!

This is known as **'fight, flight or freeze'** and it is a protective response handed down from our ancestors which keeps us safe. It's our body's way of protecting us when we feel under 'attack'. When our body recognises 'danger' it releases hormones, including adrenaline and cortisol. These push blood to our muscles, giving us the energy and strength to either 'fight' or 'run away'. Fight, flight or freeze is still useful today – but the problem is that the 'threats' we face now aren't always physical ones. In fact, more often than not they're mental and emotional threats. And that can make it hard to pin down the 'threat' we are actually facing. (It also means that surge of adrenaline isn't always very helpful when we don't have an obvious physical threat to deal with.)

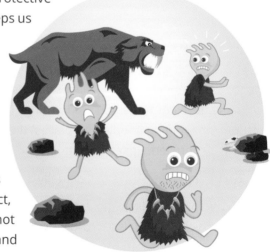

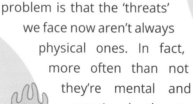

There are a number of physical sensations you may experience associated with the physiological changes in the body due to the fight, flight or freeze response.

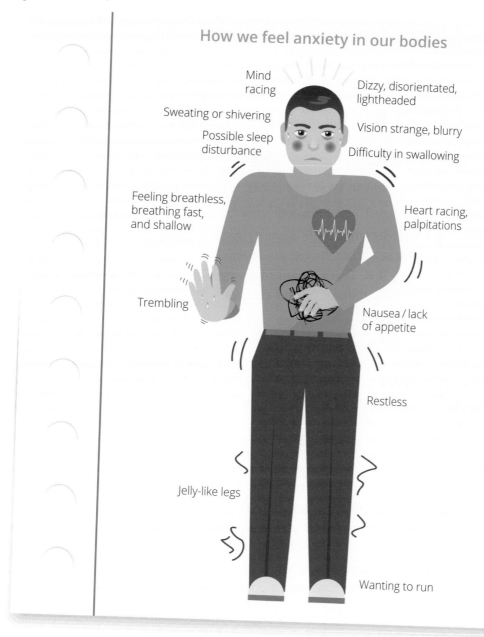

How we feel anxiety in our bodies

Mind racing

Dizzy, disorientated, lightheaded

Sweating or shivering

Vision strange, blurry

Possible sleep disturbance

Difficulty in swallowing

Feeling breathless, breathing fast, and shallow

Heart racing, palpitations

Trembling

Nausea / lack of appetite

Restless

Jelly-like legs

Wanting to run

CONFUSED? DON'T WORRY!

Read on, and we'll explain all this in more detail. Through exercises, questionnaires, and worksheets, you'll discover exactly how anxiety and worry is affecting you, and how, with a bit of practice, you can think about your worries in a different way. In fact, we can sum this up in one sentence:

If you are having problems with anxiety and worry, a lot of it is down to how you 'see' (or interpret) the 'threat'.

If that sounds a bit complicated, here's an example of how it might look:

Katie and Emily are walking down the street. They are both wearing the same pair of shoes. A girl they don't know passes them and says, 'Nice shoes!' She walks on by without another word. Katie and Emily look at each other.

'Why did she say that!?' Katie asks.

'Dunno,' says Emily. 'It was a bit random ...'

Katie thinks about it for a moment. 'That girl was being really mean,' she thinks. 'She was dissing my shoes because they're cheap. I feel really stupid now. I'll have to throw them away and buy some new ones. But I haven't got any money, so I'll just have to put up with nasty comments or stay at home ...'

Emily thinks about it for a moment. 'Wow,' she thinks, 'that girl looked pretty cool herself, and she liked my shoes. They were quite a bargain and I think they look good. And I'm right!'

So you see – two people have completely different reactions to the same event. It doesn't really matter whether the girl who said 'Nice shoes!' was being kind or sarcastic. What is important is how it made Katie and Emily feel. That's what I mean by 'interpretation'. Both Katie and Emily interpreted the girl's comments differently and consequently felt differently because of their different interpretations.

In the next few chapters, we'll have a look at this more closely. At the moment, you're probably feeling overwhelmed by your worries and can't even think about 'interpreting' them differently. That's okay. What is important is that you know that they are worries, and that it is normal to have them, and that things can be different for you. It might even help to tell someone about them.

BUT WORRY IS SO EMBARRASSING ...

Like Adam, you might think it's difficult and embarrassing to talk about your worries. That's understandable, and perfectly normal. Adam thought no one would understand him and so he didn't tell anyone. By not telling anyone, he suffered years of pain, loneliness and misery. The other big secret about anxiety and worry is that **we all experience it**. So if you choose to talk to someone – a parent, a teacher, a youth worker, a school counsellor, or a friend – they will all be able to tell you a story about their worries. Having severe anxiety DOES NOT mean you're weird, or a freak, or different to anyone else. However, it does means it's causing problems for you – so we're going to help you change that.

By reading this book, and perhaps by telling someone about your worries, you're already taking a very positive move towards sorting out your problem. Adam wasn't able to do this until he was much older (he was in his mid-30s) and that means he went on suffering right into his adulthood.

But you don't need to!

By taking control of the situation now, by understanding anxiety and worry, and by learning and using the strategies you'll discover in this book, you will feel so much better about yourself NOW.

Cognitive Behaviour Therapy (CBT)

Our **Accept-Embrace-Control** method is based on a treatment method for anxiety called Cognitive Behaviour Therapy (CBT) with a Be-Kind-To-Yourself Approach. This is a very sound, very sensible method that connects:

The things that happen in our lives, to:

The way we interpret them, to:

Our emotional, physical and behavioural responses to them.

By looking at how these are all linked, we can see how **unhelpful thinking patterns** emerge, and then explore ways we can re-think our reactions to things that happen in our lives, so that we feel better about them. Our approach is about learning new skills and testing out your reactions to the things and events that make you feel uncomfortable at the moment.

If this sounds a bit scary, it's not meant to be. We don't need to do everything all at once. In fact, taking your time to really understand and learn this approach is the best way forward.

Our approach isn't a 'quick fix', but it's a fix that will stick.

FEELING DEPRESSED

Reading this, you might think, *'My anxiety and worry is giving me such a hard time I feel really low and I don't feel I have the energy to do this.'*

I understand ... It might be the case that you're depressed as a result of your anxiety, and that's not surprising. Anxiety has a way of causing trouble that leads to depression. But if you are feeling **depressed as a result of your worries**, anxieties or OCD, there is some good news – this is likely to disappear once you've tackled your difficulties.

However, if you were depressed before you had problems with worry, anxiety or OCD, or it feels too overwhelming, then you really need to talk to someone about it (a parent, a teacher or, best of all, your local doctor). We don't cover depression as a subject in this book because it may need a different treatment to the one we're describing for worry, anxiety and OCD, but we do understand how isolating and distressing depression can be. It's a really nasty thing to have, and it can drag you down to the point where you don't feel strong enough to tackle your anxiety problem.

PLEASE DO SPEAK TO SOMEONE ABOUT DEPRESSION BEFORE IT GETS WORSE

We understand that you can be overwhelmed with sadness and loneliness when you are depressed, and this can give rise to feelings of self-harm or even suicide but **please be aware that help is out there. All you need to do is ask**. If you're feeling like this, then make an appointment to see your doctor. They will be very understanding of what you're going through, and can help you in a variety of ways.

It's hard to motivate yourself when you feel this way, but we find that by taking even very small steps at first, you will begin to notice a difference in your overall mood and approach to life.

You might also be at an age where you and your friends are drinking alcohol and maybe experimenting with drugs. We're not going to judge anyone for that, but we would just say that while it's normal to try new things in your teens, trying alcohol or drugs while you feel worried, anxious or depressed won't make your problems any better. Drink and drugs might make them disappear for a little while, but make no mistake: your problems will come back, again and again. We should also point out that alcohol and drugs actually make depression and anxiety worse! So if possible, please try to avoid drink and drugs while you're getting yourself better.

Being a teenager isn't easy!

There are a lot of good times, but bad times too. You're trying to figure out who you are, and what your place is in the world. You're dealing with complex social situations, particularly online and using social media, and you're at the mercy of hormones, peer pressure, parent pressure, school expectations and everything else! The last thing you need is an Anxiety / OCD / Worry problem, but if you see it as less of a problem and more of a challenge, you'll be taking at least one very positive step towards recovering from it.

THE KINDNESS FACTOR

Above all else – be kind to yourself. If you feel you've done something positive towards taking control of your anxiety, be proud of yourself. If you've had a bad day, don't beat yourself up. You need kindness and support. The best person to give you these things is you. I know it's difficult. But it is true. We will encourage you to treat yourself with the kindness and understanding that you deserve. This journey is hard enough without feeling down on yourself too!

Good luck with your journey, and stick with it. Adam knows, I know – and I hope you know – the end result is really going to be worth it!

CHAPTER SUMMARY

- Worry and anxiety are completely normal, and part of who we are. Worry and anxiety become a problem when they interfere a lot in our lives, and stop us doing the things we enjoy.

- Much of how worry and anxiety make us feel depends on how we interpret and react to things that might make us worried or anxious.

- By exploring how we interpret and react to things that might make us worried or anxious we can change our thoughts and reactions, and face up to our worries and anxieties, and eventually our anxiety will reduce or go away.

- Anxiety and worry is like a bully – sometimes you have to stand up to it to make it go away.

- Depression may occur as a result of anxiety, but it can disappear once you start to face your worries. Even so, if you feel depressed, it is important to tell someone and ask for help.

- Remember – always be kind to yourself during your process of recovery. You have beaten yourself up for long enough!

Chapter 17

ACCEPT

In the next few chapters, we'll be looking at how anxiety affects you and why you sometimes react in the way that you do. Our strategy here is called **'Accept'**, and what we are trying to do is get you to 'accept' that you have a problem with anxiety and understand how that problem works, so you can then begin to take charge and change it.

'Hang on a minute ...' you might think, *'... you want me to accept that I have an anxiety problem? Surely I need to REJECT anxiety?'*

Okay, I can see where you're coming from, but let's look at it this way: for a while, you've been suffering from anxiety and you've tried your best to get rid of it. As we mentioned in the last chapter, you might be doing something (using a lucky charm, counting, washing your hands, etc.) or NOT doing something (avoiding people, places and situations) to make it go away.

And let's face it. It isn't really working, is it? What you do (or don't do) to make anxiety and worry go away might have worked for a bit, but you've probably noticed that it comes back even stronger than before, or it just lurks there waiting for another opportunity to pounce.

TRY A DIFFERENT WAY OF LOOKING AT YOUR THOUGHTS?

We've talked about looking at your thoughts in a different way. We all see and interpret situations differently, So perhaps there is **another interpretation** you can tell yourself about the situation that's causing you so much anxiety? One which is much more helpful than the version currently going on inside your head at the moment. So tell me, would you sign up for a different approach – even if it meant 'accepting' your anxiety for what it is?

If so, let's delve a little deeper ...

As we've said, anxiety is an old, old condition that has been passed down to us from our cavemen ancestors. Today, we call it 'fight, flight or freeze', and while we know what that means, it isn't always easy to identify the 'threat' that prompts it. Today, it's not quite as simple as the very obvious threat of a sabre-toothed tiger!

So let's look at some up-to-date examples:

Kayleigh is 13 and has been invited to a pool party. She's never been to one before, so she is worrying about making a good impression. She knows that pictures of the event will be on Facebook, Twitter or Instagram that same day.

'All my friends will be wearing bikinis, and I look awful in mine,' she thinks. 'What should I do?'

She tries on various swimsuits, but nothing feels right. As the day of the party approaches she feels sick to her stomach and gets hot and sweaty just thinking about it. On the day of the party itself, she wakes up and thinks, 'I just can't do it. I can't go.' And so she rings her friend and makes the excuse that she's sick. Her friend is upset, but the pool party goes ahead anyway and everyone has a good time. No one really cares what anyone else is wearing. Kayleigh doesn't know this, of course, because she's at home in her bedroom, feeling upset.

So, was the story Kayleigh told herself about the party (that she would be judged negatively by her friends and other people) accurate? Was it helpful? Was she right to think in the way she did, or was her anxiety telling her how she should react?

Is there anything she could have told herself that would have made it better for herself? What could she have done differently?

Let's look at another example:

James is 16, and has always been the clever kid at school. But in his final year, he has developed worries around his exams. He feels it is important that he gets good grades; he also feels there is pressure from his school and his parents to do well. The thought of not doing well makes James feel sick, shaky and sweaty. He finds it hard to sleep and his revision is suffering as a result. He finds ways to avoid doing the work he needs to do to get the good grades. During exam week James avoids going into some exams, saying he doesn't feel well. He attends other exams, but leaves halfway through. When his results arrive, he has done a lot less well than anyone expected.

So was the story James told himself about the exams (that he would fail, and let himself and his family down) accurate? Was it helpful? Was he right to think in the way he did, or was his anxiety telling him how he should react?

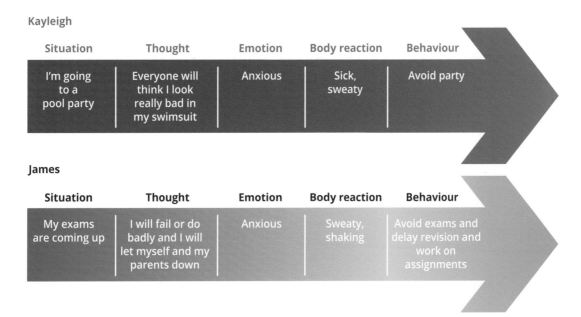

Figure 1: *How we interpret events affects our emotional, physiological and behavioural responses.*

Is there anything he could have told himself that would have made it better for himself? What could he have done differently?

In both cases, anxiety over upcoming events caused Kayleigh and James to avoid them. And in both cases, they lost out. Below is a diagram which sets out the sequence of events for both Kayleigh and James, and how they felt:

Now, let's see if we can come up with a better story for James and Kayleigh.

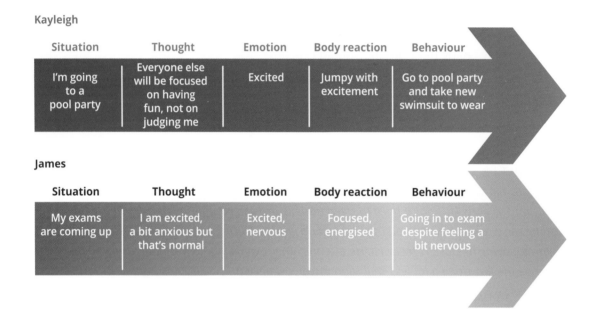

Kayleigh				
Situation	**Thought**	**Emotion**	**Body reaction**	**Behaviour**
I'm going to a pool party	Everyone else will be focused on having fun, not on judging me	Excited	Jumpy with excitement	Go to pool party and take new swimsuit to wear

James				
Situation	**Thought**	**Emotion**	**Body reaction**	**Behaviour**
My exams are coming up	I am excited, a bit anxious but that's normal	Excited, nervous	Focused, energised	Going in to exam despite feeling a bit nervous

Figure 2: *How we interpret events affects our emotional, physiological and behavioural responses.*

So you see, there is a different story to be told by James and Kayleigh and even if they're a bit worried, apprehensive and anxious, this isn't going to put them off doing what they want to do.

Your major worries

Let's go through a few questions to find out what your main worries are, and how anxiety is affecting your life. Have a think and if it's helpful, write in the boxes below:

WHAT DO YOU THINK ARE YOUR MAIN WORRIES?

_____

_____

_____

_____

_____

_____

_____

WORRY AND ANXIETY AFFECTS MY LIFE IN THESE WAYS ...
(THINGS YOU ARE AVOIDING OR THINGS THAT YOU HAVE TO DO THAT YOU WISH YOU DIDN'T NEED TO DO).

_____

_____

_____

_____

_____

_____

_____

WHEN YOU HAVE THESE WORRIES WHAT EMOTIONS DO YOU FEEL,
AND HOW DO YOU FEEL IN YOUR BODY?

_____

_____

_____

_____

_____

_____

HOW WOULD I LIKE TO CHANGE MY 'STORY' OR GIVE THE SITUATION A
MORE USEFUL AND HELPFUL INTERPRETATION?

_____

_____

_____

_____

_____

_____

_____

_____

Now you've filled this in, and had time to reflect on it, let's look more closely at how your situation has become increasingly difficult. It might be that you feel very muddled and confused about it all, so let's break it down into stages. The reason for doing this is to help you see the link between the situation and your thoughts, feelings, bodily reactions and behaviour.

WHEN DID YOU LAST EXPERIENCE YOUR PROBLEM?
WHERE WERE YOU?

DESCRIBE WHAT HAPPENED:

WHAT WAS GOING THROUGH YOUR HEAD AT THE TIME? WHAT DID YOU THINK
WAS THE WORST THING THAT COULD POSSIBLY HAPPEN?

WHAT EMOTIONS DID YOU FEEL? (ANGRY / SAD / WORRIED / FEARFUL / ASHAMED ETC.)

_____

_____

_____

_____

HOW DID YOU FEEL IN YOUR BODY? (SWEATY? SHAKY? SICK? JITTERY? ETC.)

_____

_____

_____

_____

HOW DID YOU REACT - WHAT DID YOU DO, OR NOT DO?

_____

_____

_____

_____

WHAT HAPPENED AS A RESULT?

_____

_____

_____

_____

JOINING IT ALL UP

Hopefully, you might now be starting to see how your worries and reactions join up to create anxious periods. We call this an **'unhelpful anxiety trap'** and if we step back from a situation we can see patterns of **'unhelpful thinking'** emerge. 'Unhelpful thinking' is a way of describing types of interpretations that are very unhelpful and aren't usually true, which keep us trapped in the anxiety trap.

Of course, anxiety doesn't always work in a logical order. Sometimes you just have a feeling in your stomach that something is 'wrong' and you don't know why. That's very normal, and if it's happened to you, it is worth asking yourself these questions:

- What was the situation you were in when you started feeling uncomfortable? or
- What were you thinking about when you started feeling uncomfortable? or
- What were you doing (or avoiding doing) at the time?

Think very hard about these, and see if you can write down some answers in the box below ...

To finish this chapter, let's remind ourselves that **accepting** we have worries and anxieties doesn't mean we're giving in to them. In fact, we're doing the opposite. But if we don't accept our situation, and we carry on **fighting** our worries and anxieties, we give them **power** over us.

So **accepting** your state of mind and emotional state means you are **owning** it for what it is.

CHAPTER SUMMARY

- The best way to begin tackling our anxiety problem is to accept that we have a problem in the first place.

- 'Fight, flight or freeze' is the body's way of reacting to 'threat'. In some situations it can be useful; in others, it can cause worry and anxiety. When humans first experienced 'fight, flight or freeze' the threats they experienced may have seemed very different, but really, the fears they created of being rejected by their tribe for not being fast / strong / quick enough were very similar.

- How we react to 'threats' either increases or decreases our anxieties and worries.

- Anxieties, worries and our reactions to them join up to create anxious periods we call 'anxiety traps'.

- We can learn to tell ourselves another story or have another interpretation for the situation in which we react to 'threat'.

Chapter 18

Are You Falling into Thinking Traps?

In the last chapter we saw how worry and anxiety create an anxiety trap and push along a process which leaves you feeling terrible, forcing you to try to do something about your worry and anxiety that generally doesn't work.

THE WORRY WHEEL

Another way of looking at this anxiety trap is by using the diagram of a 'vicious cycle' of worry, or what we call a 'Worry Wheel'. If you've ever looked inside an old clock or a watch, you'll have noticed that it uses little cogs, or wheels that connect with each other as they go round.

Worry and anxiety work in the same way. Have a look at the diagram below:

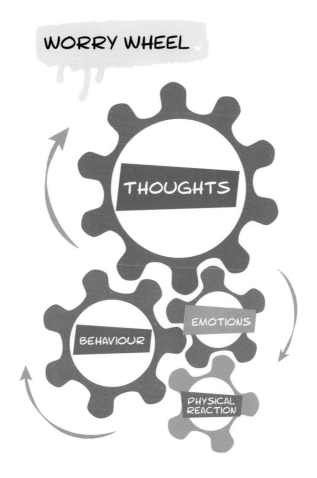

You'll see how your thoughts (at the top) push round the Emotions wheel, then the Physical Reaction wheel, then the Behaviour wheel, until they're all spinning at once – and you're feeling about as bad as you can possibly feel!

Let's see how this works in the case of Amy:

Amy is often the last person out of her house each morning as her parents start work early. They have given her the responsibility of locking up. She worries terribly about leaving an electrical appliance (kettle, hairdryer, laptop etc.) switched on in case it overheats and causes a fire. This makes her so anxious that she spends about 30 minutes each morning checking that every appliance is turned off and every plug is unplugged. This causes her to be frequently late for college.

Let's have a look at the diagram:

Although Amy has only ever read about house fires (never having experienced one) and could probably switch off all the items in five minutes, the anxiety she experiences at the mere thought of a fire forces her to check, check and check again before she can leave the house.

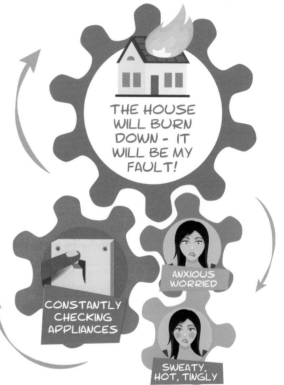

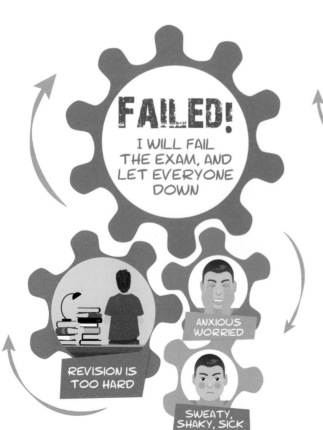

Remember James and the school exam? The one he was avoiding because he didn't want to fail and let everyone down? Let's have a look at his Worry Wheel:

At the top we have his thought ('I will fail the exam, and let everyone down') which pushes along his anxiety. In his body he feels sick, sweaty and shaky every time he thinks about the exam, which in turn drives the final cog, which is about James finding revision so hard that eventually he seeks ways to avoid the exam altogether.

Below is a diagram of the Worry Wheel. Have another look at James's and Amy's wheels, above, and fill in the gaps with your own view of how your worry works:

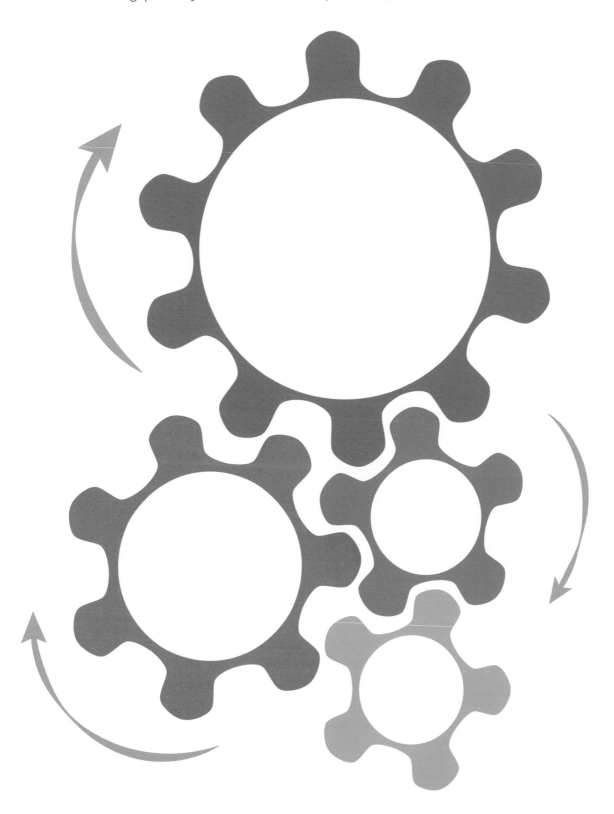

THOUGHTS ABOUT THOUGHTS

I mentioned the phrase 'mere thought' above. Let's have a look at thoughts for a moment. It's estimated that we have between 50,000 to 70,000 thoughts a day. That's a lot of thinking to pack into one brain! These are what we call 'automatic thoughts'. Some of these will be intrusive thoughts. They are uncontrollable and cause us a lot of distress. These are the ones that stick around a bit longer, and which can cause trouble when you take them seriously, and attach 'importance' to them. Everyone has these uncontrollable intrusive thoughts; it's what you think or do about them which counts.

We also have another set of thoughts that we're less aware of. We call these **Rules** or **Assumptions**, and **Core Beliefs**. These determine how we see ourselves, others and our place in the world. These core beliefs inform our assumptions about the world, and set the rules that we live by day-to-day, sometimes for our whole lives, without ever bothering to challenge them. These can include rules like:

- It's important to be liked by others, **otherwise** it means I am not a good enough person.
- It's important to be careful with your belongings, **otherwise** it means you are careless.
- It's important never to be late, **otherwise** you look like a lazy person.

On the surface, some of these rules look like good ones to live by. However, if you pay a lot of attention to them, they could lead to worry and anxiety, particularly if you are feeling stressed that you might lose something important, or that you go out of your way to please everybody, or that you get upset if you or someone else is late for something that's not so important.

These rules can be useful guidelines, but although we call them 'rules', and often live by them like they were laws, they aren't really rules. They're just guidelines by which we like to live our lives – and we can change them whenever we like. This is useful for us to remember, especially when these 'rules' have become so fixed that they cause upset and disturbance in our daily life.

Also, there are Core Beliefs. These are more fixed statements about what we believe about the world, our place in it, and other people. It can include things like:

- The world is dangerous
- I am unlovable
- Other people are difficult
- I'm never wrong

We all hold strong beliefs about ourselves and the world, which we often hang on to all our lives. But these beliefs can become very fixed, and very hard to shake off if they are causing us difficulties. If we see the world as dangerous, we might never leave our home town. But if we see the world as a place of wonder we realise it is there to be explored, despite possible dangers. We might think other people are careless and incompetent, and that only we can do things properly. Or perhaps we're happy to allow other people to take responsibility for things, believing they know more than us.

We all hold beliefs, with different levels of strength. And as we've seen, it's not the thoughts we have on a daily basis, but the **importance we give them** which often comes from core beliefs. If you believe the world is a dangerous place and you're happy to stay in your neighbourhood and never go anywhere else, then fine. But if you long to visit friends or relatives in another country and you can't because of a belief that something will happen to you, **then this is what we'd call 'Unhelpful Thinking'**. If your worries and anxieties are strong and regular, and you feel panicky or uncomfortable every time you think about or experience the trigger which sets them off, these are indications that something is wrong.

Let's look at these automatic thoughts, rules and Core Beliefs in terms of a volcano. Inside the 'mountain', at the bottom, lie the Core Beliefs. When these start rumbling and boiling, they activate the Rules and Assumptions and these eventually push the 'lava' of your automatic and intrusive thoughts sky-high!

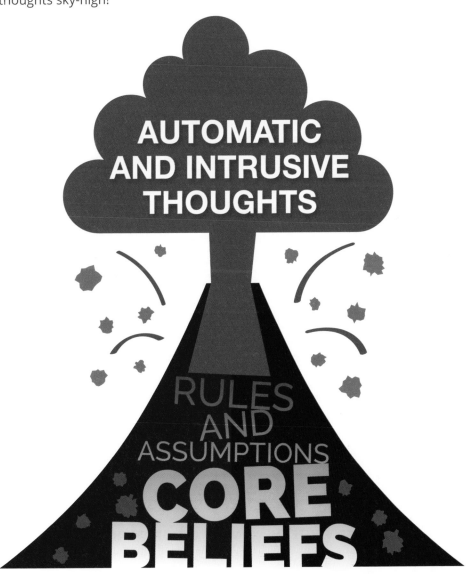

THINKING TRAPS

The Unhelpful Thinking Patterns that we've described above, which we can also call '**Thinking Traps**', can apply to any of the thoughts we've described above. This means that they can bring trouble into your life if you pay them too much attention. Some of them include:

GLOOM-AND-DOOMING or WORST CASE SCENARIO: Thinking the worst-case scenario about every event, no matter how minor. 'If I leave the house without checking the window someone will definitely break into the house.'

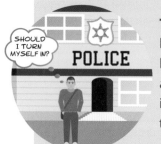

THINKING INTO EXISTENCE[1]: That having a thought means it is more likely to happen, or it means that thinking about the action is as bad as actually doing it. 'Because I had this thought it means that I am more likely to hurt someone, or that I must really want to hurt someone.'

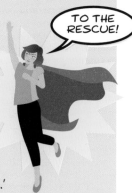

ME TO THE RESCUE! Believing you are 100 per cent responsible or have an increased responsibility for things, discounting the fact that other people may share responsibility.[2] 'I am the only person responsible for making sure the window is secure, therefore if anyone breaks in through the open window it will be 100 per cent my fault.'

BLAMING AND SHAMING: Thinking that everything is your fault, even when you couldn't have had anything to do with it. 'My team lost, I'm a jinx – I shouldn't have been at the match!'

REASONING WITH WORRIES: When you try to reason or argue with your worries in order to make them see sense, but you can never win! 'If I don't go to the party then people will think I'm a loser, but if I do go, I might say something weird or strange and people will think I'm stupid.'

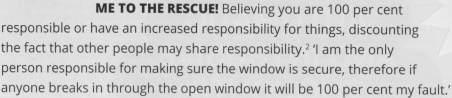

BARGAINING WITH WORRIES: This is the OCD version of Reasoning With Worries. 'If I do this ritual, it will be the last time that I do it!'

BLACK-AND-WHITE THINKING or ALL OR NOTHING THINKING: You categorise experiences or things one way or another, often as good or bad, with no in-between. 'If I don't pass this exam with an A, I've failed.'

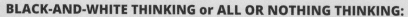

FORTUNE TELLING: Thinking you can predict the future, or living as if the future has happened. 'I know exactly what will happen if I go to this party ...'

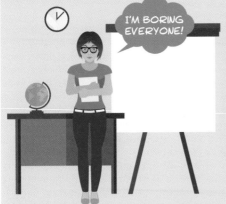

JUMPING TO CONCLUSIONS: Making a judgement, usually negative, even when there is little or no evidence for it. 'This person hasn't texted me back or messaged me on Facebook so they must be ignoring me ...'

'SHOULD BE' and 'OUGHT TO BE': Thinking things HAVE to be a certain way, or people (including you) SHOULD behave in a particular way. 'I SHOULD get 100 per cent in every test.' 'People OUGHT TO BE friendly all the time.' 'People SHOULD text back immediately.'

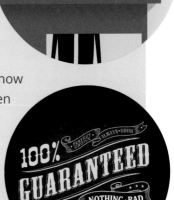

GUARANTEES ABOUT THE FUTURE: Needing everything to be guaranteed or the outcome of events to be known, despite that being impossible. 'I need to know 100 per cent that something bad won't happen in the future.'

EMOTIONAL REASONING: Basing things on how you feel, rather than basing them on reality. 'I just FEEL that something bad will happen.'

MASTERY OF THE UNIVERSE: Believing you have control over events or outcomes, that you cannot actually influence. 'If I do all these chores right, then my family will be safe.' This can sometimes be known as MAGICAL THINKING in its extreme form. 'If I don't touch the light switch six times then my grandmother in Australia will become ill or die.'

MIND READING: Believing that you know what other people are thinking, despite having no evidence for it. 'I know that my colleague thinks I am stupid.'

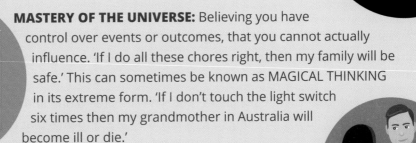

You may be able to see that your own worry lies within one or more of these thinking traps. If so, fill in the box below which will help you to see what your worries are, which thinking traps they apply to, and why:

MY WORRY IS ...

_____

_____

_____

_____

THE THINKING TRAPS THAT APPLY TO MY WORRY ARE ...

_____

_____

_____

_____

Let's have a look at how these might apply in real life:

Four teenagers – Sam, Ellie, Bryony and Jack – are all worriers in different ways. One Saturday night they all receive the same text from their friend, Martyn. It says, 'Are you at home tonight?'

Sam is a Worst-Case Scenario thinker. 'Oh no!' _he thinks._ 'Martyn's gonna tell everyone at school on Monday that I was home on Saturday night, and the whole year will be laughing at me. It's the end of my life!!!'

Ellie is a Rescuer. 'Oh no!' _she thinks._ 'Martyn must be at home, with nothing to do. He wants to go out, and I really don't, but I'll have to go now because if I don't he will get upset and it'll ALL BE MY FAULT!!!!'

Bryony is a Mind Reader. 'Oh no!' _she thinks,_ 'Martyn wants to go out, and I don't, but I just know what he'll think of me if I don't go along to that terrible cafe in town – that I'm a loser for staying in on a Saturday night.'

Jack is a 'Should Be / Ought to Be' kind of person. 'Oh no!' _he thinks._ 'Martyn should've explained much more clearly what he means. He ought to send another text so that I completely understand what he's asking me here. But he'll expect me to text back straightaway. I suppose I should be out on a Saturday night anyway.'

And so on. Can you see how this works? Martyn was just asking a simple question, yet his four friends turned it into something much more complicated because they allowed their thoughts to act like bullies, pushing them into a certain way of thinking.

But thoughts aren't really bullies. Thoughts don't have minds of their own. **They're just thoughts!** And if we **accept** them for what they are – 'just thoughts' – then we can change them. Now do you see why 'accepting' our thoughts is a good thing, not a bad thing?

Remember – we all have unwelcome thoughts. Kings, queens, presidents, prime ministers, celebrities, sportsmen and women, teachers, police officers, and even your friends all have unwelcome thoughts. Every single person experiences life events that are beyond their control. To manage anxiety, worry, and OCD, you have to ACCEPT this as fact. When you do, you'll start to feel much better!

Before we move on to the **EMBRACE** section, have another read through everything we've looked at so far and, if possible, write down the worries and experiences you've had that have been beyond your control. Writing them down helps you to understand them. And sharing them – even if it's only with yourself – can be very helpful!

TALK ABOUT IT ...

As we've said, your worries could be about anything. Today, bullying – especially online – affects a lot of people, all over the world. Teenagers who use social media to upset, intimidate and generally stress out others are just as bullying as if they'd physically hit their victims in the face. The worry caused by online bullying can creep into other areas of our lives, making us feel miserable and anxious, depressed, and even suicidal.

If this has ever happened to you, and made you feel like this, you should **tell someone**. Although there are many things you can do alone to manage your worries, you need other people to help you overcome bullying of this kind. As ever, be kind to yourself.

Try to accept that you feel this way without judging yourself for it, and remember that, no matter how intense the feeling is, **it is not permanent**. If you accept this, then you can choose to do something different in that moment. I don't mean trying to avoid the feeling (which isn't the best approach) but saying, 'It's okay to feel bad now, but I won't feel this bad forever.' Give yourself some space and some time to do something just for you. It could be something simple like going for a walk or playing a game, reading a book, listening to music or making some of your favourite food. In other words, try to be kind to yourself.

CHAPTER SUMMARY

- Our worrying thoughts can push round a 'Worry Wheel' which gives us anxious and uncomfortable feelings in our bodies. Sometimes, it feels like the only thing we can do to make the thoughts and feelings go away is do certain things (like counting rituals, or turning switches on and off). Sometimes we feel compelled not to do certain things; we may even avoid going to certain places or doing things that we would normally enjoy doing.

- Everyone has strange / silly / weird / uncomfortable and uncontrollable thoughts, images, doubts and feelings that we call 'intrusions'. If we focus on them and worry about them, it gives them power to disrupt our lives. If we remember that they are just passing thoughts, it can take their power away.

- We all live by Rules and Core Beliefs. These are part of who we are and define how we see and experience the world. Some of these interpretations can be really unhelpful and we call them 'Thinking Traps'. If we fall into our personal Thinking Traps we can believe things about ourselves, our friends and the world which simply aren't true. But if we identify them for what they are, we can start to change them. Just like our rules and core beliefs, intrusions can fall into thinking traps too. Identifying the thinking traps that our core beliefs, rules and intrusions fall into can help us go on to change them.

Chapter 19

EMBRACE

In the next couple of chapters we're going to look at ways we can challenge and overcome our worries and anxieties. We've called these techniques 'Embrace' because I'm going to ask you to face up to your worries and embrace them!

WHY DO I WANT TO 'EMBRACE' MY WORRIES? I HATE THEM!

When you embrace your worries you will make them non-threatening. When you take the decision to face up to your worries and anxieties, you get all the power. Your worries can't ever creep up on you if you're embracing them!

STILL SOUND A BIT WEIRD?

Well, maybe – but in the last section I told you that you would 'accept' your worries and not fight them, and that's what you've done!

Before we fully embrace our worries, we need to spend a little time weighing them up, and seeing if what they're telling us is really true. Doing this is a bit like being a lawyer in a courtroom trial, or a detective investigating a crime; you look at all the evidence and see which version of events is closest to the truth.

THE 'TWO HANDS' TEST

To do this, we're going to use a technique called the **'Two Hands Theory'**. This is based on the fact that **there are always two sides to every story. For example, we might think, 'On the one hand, I'm disappointed I got such a low grade, maybe I'm not as clever as I thought. But on the other hand, we can think, 'I didn't put that much effort in to revising. Next time, I'll make sure I have more time to revise and I'll do a lot better.'** We're aiming to find the story that is most helpful to us. So let's see what happened to Mira after she posted a picture of herself online ...

Mira is 15, and she sometimes posts selfies on Instagram. But one day, instead of the usual 'likes' and positive comments, she received a whole stream of horrible remarks on her appearance, clothing and hair. Mira didn't recognise any of the 'haters' but she imagined they were people from school who were being mean to her behind her back. She decided that, far from being liked by other students as she had thought, she must actually be really unpopular.

This makes life difficult for Mira because she feels like she doesn't know who to trust among her friends any more. Every time she sees a group of them, she feels sick and walks round the corner to avoid them. Her friends are now wondering why she's ignoring them.

Okay, let's see what happens when we apply the Two Hands Theory to Mira's story.

On the One Hand, Mira's thoughts are telling her that people at school don't like her. Why? Because she has received some horrible comments online.

BUT...

On the Other Hand, Mira might realise that she can't prove it's her friends who have made the comments. It could be random strangers, 'trolls' who just want to annoy someone. If someone she knows HAS posted the comments, then they're not worth knowing any more.

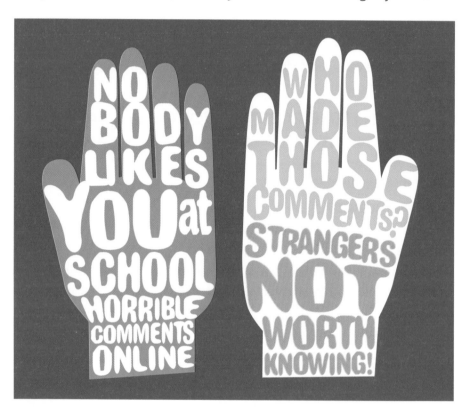

Let's have a look at Zak's story as another example:

Zak is 13, and suffers with horrible OCD. He gets intrusive thoughts about harming his little brother, Ethan, who is 6. This really bothers Zak, because he thinks it might mean that one day he will become a murderer. To avoid the thought and keep his brother safe, Zak carries out a 'compulsion', which is to do everything he can to avoid being around Ethan. It means he can never play with his little brother. This is really sad, because Ethan wants to play with his big brother and Zak's parents think he is being 'moody'. But Zak is too frightened of his thoughts to tell anyone about them, because they might think he could turn into a murderer too!

So we can see how this is really difficult for Zak. Let's now play detective, and apply the Two Hands Theory to his story.

On the One Hand, Zak's thoughts are telling him that he is a danger to other people. Why? Because he has bad thoughts about harming his little brother, and he feels he must treat these thoughts seriously.

BUT...

On the Other Hand, Zak might realise that he is a sensitive, caring person who is worried about being a danger to others. In reality, he is not a danger at all. Hurting someone is the last thing he would ever do!

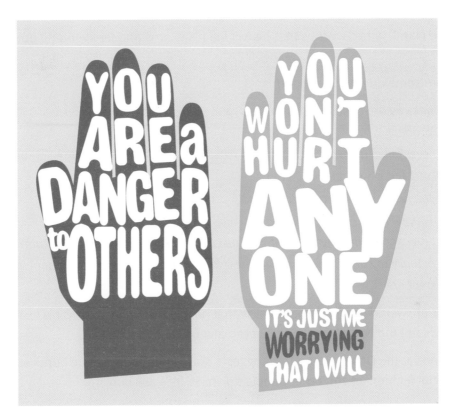

Which do you think is true? Well, let's look at the evidence by putting Zak in the witness box and asking him some questions ...

Q: Zak, have you ever attacked Ethan?

Zak: No.

Q: Zak, have you ever attacked anyone?

Zak: No! I hate the thought of violence ...

Q: Have you ever made a plan to attack anyone?

Zak: Never.

Q: Has a doctor ever examined you, and diagnosed that you are a danger to others?

Zak: No!

Q: Do you enjoy thoughts of harming people?

Zak: No, I hate them!

To me, it looks pretty convincing. Unless Zak is a very good liar, which I doubt, I think it is safe to say that Zak is NOT a danger to anyone. His problem is that he **worries** that he is a danger to people. So I would say that the 'Other Hand' explanation is the correct one.

Do you agree? And if so, do you see the difference between 'the one hand' and 'the other hand'? Let's put someone else's worries 'on trial' to see where the truth lies …

Remember James, who was worried about failing his exams? He's a clever kid who feels under pressure (mainly from himself) to do well. His worries are disturbing his revision and he's not even sure if he can face walking into the exam room.

On the **One Hand**, James worries that he will fail his exams and let everyone down, especially himself.

Let's ask him some questions about this.

Q: Do you think you are clever enough to pass your exams?
James: *Yes, probably.*
Q: Have you ever failed an exam?
James: *Well, no. But it'd be terrible if I did.*
Q: Couldn't you just take the exam again?
James: *Yes, I suppose so – if I had to.*
Q: Have you ever known anyone's life to fall to pieces because they've failed an exam?
James: *No, actually my dad failed his driving test four times, but he kept going until he passed. Now he's a great driver.*

If James has answered truthfully, he'll realise that he has the ability to pass his exams, and even if he doesn't it's not the end of the world. He can always take them again.

Now, let's look at the **Other Hand**. This suggests that James believes one hundred per cent it is important to not let himself and other people down. So let's ask him:

Q: James, do you think that maybe you worry a bit too much?
James: *Yes, probably.*
Q: Do you think it will be the end of the world if you didn't pass an exam first time?
James: *Well … no. But I wouldn't like it.*
Q: Do you feel anxious in your body?
James: *Yes, regularly.*
Q: Do you think that worrying about passing your exams will actually help you to pass?
James: *No, it won't!*

If James has answered these questions truthfully, he'll realise that his problem is about the worry of failing his exams, rather than the likelihood of it actually happening.

Let's look at another example:

Carla, 15, has OCD and experiences thoughts about not leaving water running in the house in case it causes a flood. She thinks that if it happens, she will be responsible for it, causing her family to suffer. Before she goes out she has to check every tap, and the shower, to make sure they're all turned off tightly. This often makes her late for school and drives her 11-year-old sister Bethany annoyed because she isn't strong enough to turn the tap on when she wants to brush her teeth!

So, on the **One Hand**, Carla worries that she is careless and could cause a flood. She tries to make sure this doesn't happen by checking and turning off taps.

We could ask Carla a few questions to help us work out the truth:

1) Has she ever experienced a flood? Probably not, but if she has …
2) Was it so bad that it destroyed her life? Probably not.
3) Has it happened to anyone she knows? Probably not.
4) Has she read about flooding, or seen TV pictures of it? Yes, she has.
5) Was it terrible? Yes, it was at the time, but everything was fixed up in the end – and besides, flooding on this scale was caused by bad weather, not a tap!

If Carla has answered these questions truthfully she'll realise that such flooding is rare, and if it does happen it's not nearly as bad as she imagines. So there is little evidence for the One Hand point of view.

Now, let's look at the **Other Hand**. This suggests that Carla feels responsible for things that might go wrong, and that she believes it is important to be careful or something bad might happen. So let's ask her:

Q: Do you worry too much?
Carla: Yes, probably.
Q: Do you feel responsible for making sure lots of other things don't go wrong?
Carla: Yes, I do.
Q: Do you get anxious feelings in your body?
Carla: Yes, a lot of the time.
Q: Will turning the tap off tightly 100 per cent guarantee there will never, ever be a flood?
Carla: Well … no, it won't!

If Carla has answered these questions truthfully, she'll realise that her problem is about the **worry** of a flood happening, rather than it **actually** happening.

Your worries on trial

Okay, now you're going to put your own worries on trial to help you find out the truth ... Using the boxes, write down your worry problem and then put it 'on trial' to see the evidence stack up, for and against.

ON THE 'ONE HAND' MY PROBLEM IS ...

WHAT WAYS AM I LIVING MY LIFE BECAUSE OF THIS:
(i.e. what am I doing to make sure it doesn't happen, and what will I need to do in the future to continue to prevent it coming true?)

EVIDENCE FOR THIS POSITION BEING TRUE:

ON THE 'OTHER HAND' MY PROBLEM IS THAT I WORRY THAT ...

_____

_____

_____

_____

WAYS I COULD LIVE MY LIFE IF THIS WAS ONLY A WORRY PROBLEM RATHER
THAN IT BEING REAL:

_____

_____

_____

EVIDENCE FOR THIS POSITION BEING TRUE:

_____

_____

_____

_____

_____

_____

_____

BASED ON THE EVIDENCE, WHICH POSITION DO YOU THINK IS MORE LIKELY
TO BE TRUE?

So, which position do you feel lies closest to the truth? My guess is that it's the Other Hand – that this is really a worry problem. Now you're beginning to see that the problem is one of **interpretation, not reality**.

All this is fine – but just because you know it's a problem of worry, not reality, it doesn't make your worries feel any less real, does it!?

Of course it doesn't, and that's perfectly normal.

I've never met anyone in therapy with me who hasn't had doubts like that. If your worries are making you feel sweaty, panicky, sick or shaky, those are very real sensations. And worry doesn't go away so easily.

EMBRACE YOUR WORRY BIG TIME!

So what should we do about it? Well, here comes the 'embrace' bit …! The way to overcome your worry – actually, the ONLY way to overcome your worry – is to embrace it. Go right to the source of your worry, grab it to you and hold on. And keep doing it until you've embraced it so hard it can't take any more. That's what makes worries disappear. The more you do this, the more you'll see your worries for what they are – normal thoughts that can just drift away like the tens of thousands of other thoughts you have every day.

Here are some examples for you:

• If you're frightened of dogs, find one you can stroke.
• If you're frightened of speaking in public, join the school debating society.
• If you're worried about flooding, turn on a tap and leave the house for 15 minutes.
• If you don't like confined spaces, join a caving club.
• And so on … do the exact opposite of what your worry tells you to do, which is to run away!

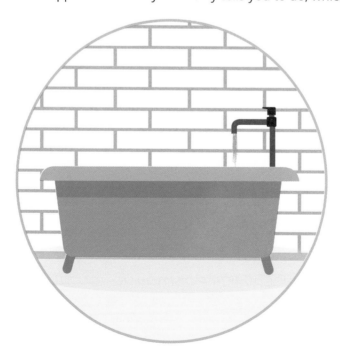

Now, I'm not a mind reader but I can probably take a guess at what you're thinking right now ... *'There's NO WAY I can do THAT!!!'*

Am I right? Yeah, thought so!

You're thinking, 'It's the fear of THAT which is giving me all these problems.' Well, yes and no. As we've seen, it's not the thing itself that is causing problems, but the worry behind it. And the only way to conquer the worry is to do the thing the worry doesn't want you to do.

Trust me, it works.

Before we look at this in more detail, let's just think about what you've been doing to push your worries away up to now. When you come up against your worry (like a dog, a spider, a trip to the pool, or whatever) your anxiety level shoots right up. So you either run away from the situation, avoid it, or carry out a ritual or a safety behaviour (counting, checking, etc.) to make yourself feel better. Okay, your anxiety level drops and you do feel better – until the next time, when you have to do the same thing again until the feeling goes away. And again, and again and again. So you're not really getting anywhere because you still have to avoid the things making you anxious, or carry out your safety behaviours.

Below is a graph to show this:

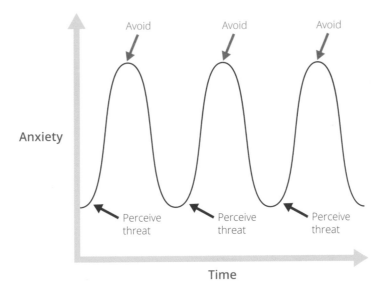

Figure 3: Avoidance of threat.

DECREASING THE THREAT

But if you embrace the worry instead of running away from it, the threat will seem less and less worrying over time. For example, if you're frightened of dogs and you always run away when you see one, the way to solve this is to stand close to a dog you can trust. You may not like it at first, but if you keep seeing the dog and eventually start to pat it, I guarantee that within a few weeks you'll be perfectly happy around that dog. Maybe you'll even take him out for walks. Who knows ... maybe you'll even start to want a dog of your own!

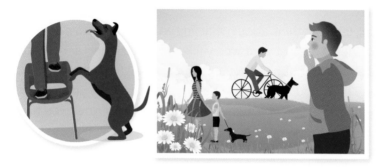

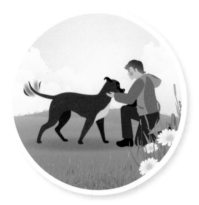
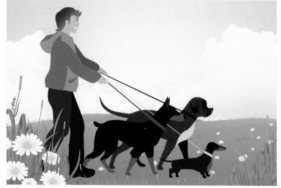

Below is a graph to show how this works:

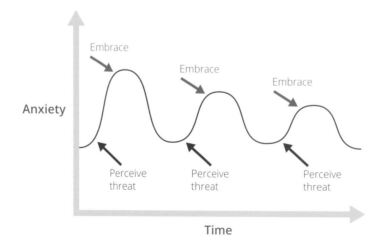

Figure 4: Exposure to threat / habituation of anxiety.

Still not convinced? Okay, let's have a look at this story ...

Harry is leaving college and wants to go into Forestry Management. He is taken on by a timber company and is sent out with two lumberjacks to see how they work. On his first day, they decide to prank him by telling him to hold up a large, low-hanging branch of a tree which, they explain, is in danger of falling down because it is so old. Then they walk off and leave him all alone, supporting the branch. A walker comes along and asks Harry why he's propping up the branch.

'Because it will fall down otherwise,' he replies.

'How do you know?' the walker replies.

'Because that's what I've been told.'

Instead of laughing at him and carrying on his way, the walker suggests that Harry takes one hand away from the branch. Harry's not keen, because he's been told to hold it up and he doesn't want to lose his job on the first day. Neither does he want the branch to fall on his head. However, he takes the plunge and tentatively removes one hand. The branch doesn't fall.

'Okay,' says the walker, 'why don't you take your other hand away now?'

'No way,' Harry replies, 'this might be the hand that stops the whole thing crashing down.'

'Or,' replies the walker, 'that might not happen at all. It might just be that you're worried it will happen. Maybe you should try it and see ...?'

Carefully, Harry removes the other hand. The tree remains as steady as it has done for the past 200 years. Harry looks at it.

'It's old,' he said. 'It could still just fall down.'

'In that case,' says the walker, 'why don't you swing on the branch?'

Harry is very nervous. Of course he is. Instead of supporting the branch he is now going to do the exact opposite and try to make it fall down! He grabs the branch with both hands and begins to swing. Surprise, surprise – nothing happens!

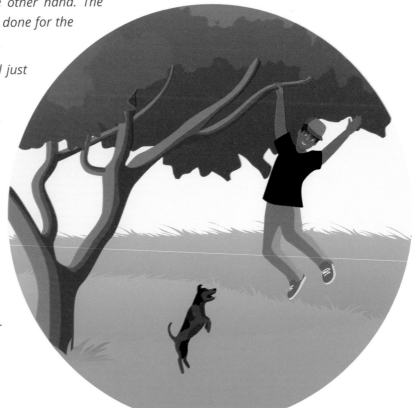

JUST SEE WHAT HAPPENS

The lesson is that you never know until you try, and it's the same with anxiety. You have to jump on the branch to see what happens – because you don't actually know. Your worry is telling you one thing, and you are living like that is the reality – but actually you don't know if that is true. There are no guarantees in life, and you have to deal with uncertainty in almost everything. So what's stopping you from at least giving it a go? You will still feel anxious, unsure and worried, but it will get easier every time.

If you're worried about something for a reason, try this experiment. Get a piece of paper and write down or sketch the worry in front of you. For example, let's say it's a dog ...

Now, here are ten stick figures lined up in front of the dog.

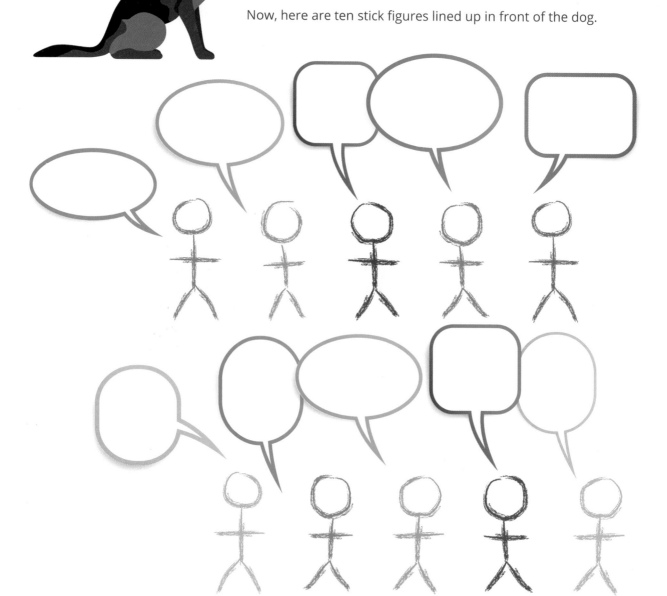

In the speech bubbles above their heads, you can write what each person is thinking about when when they see the dog. They'll probably all think slightly different thoughts – just like people react to things in different ways in real life.

Done it? There is no one 'right' way of looking at something, and if you have a thought about something that you don't like, you can always jump into someone else's shoes in the picture and have their thought instead.

So instead of sticking with your worry over a situation, try to see it in a different way. **Tell yourself a different story.** Like Harry and the tree, you never know until you try!

Worrying about what **might or might not** happen is the problem, not what will or won't happen in reality.

In the next chapter, we're going to take this strategy a bit further by setting up some **experiments** to test it out. By now, you will know what your worry is all about, so take a deep breath and get ready to walk towards it. DON'T WORRY – I won't make you do it all at once! That wouldn't be very helpful, so instead we'll take it step-by-step.

CHAPTER SUMMARY

- Don't push your worries and anxieties away. Go up to them and embrace them.
- We are beginning to see that it's not the 'thing' itself which is causing you problems, it's you **worrying** about it.
- Examine your worries and anxieties using the 'Two Hands' method. Which of the 'hands' is closest to the truth about your worries? When you examine the evidence you will see whether what you're experiencing is actually a worry problem ... If it is, then we can do something to help you stop worrying.
- The way to tackle worry and anxiety is to do the very thing worry and anxiety doesn't want you to do – which is to go forward and embrace it. By doing this, your worries and anxieties will get smaller, and go on getting smaller.

Chapter 20

Testing It All Out

Okay, this is where we're going to put all the theory into practice. You can do it!

If you have studied science at school or college, you'll know that we set up experiments in order to test out certain ideas or theories. We're not looking for the 'right' answer (because if we were, that would defeat the whole point of the experiment!) All we're doing is seeing what happens, and learning from what we discover. Over centuries, scientists who have carried out experiments have come up with ideas and inventions that have changed the world.

YOU ARE THE SCIENTIST ...

So now it's time to change **your** world! You are now the scientist and your laboratory is the world around you.

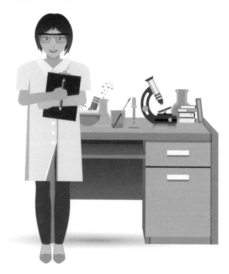

Inside the lab are jars containing your worries and anxieties. During the experiment, you will open the lids of these jars to find out what REALLY exists inside them. That may feel scary, but it is the only way to find out exactly what is going on for you. And by carrying out these experiments you are showing the same kind of **courage** and pioneering spirit as those brave scientists who found cures for many illnesses, and even managed to send people up into space. Before you start your first experiment, check in with how you're feeling, both in your mind and body. Write down some words in the box below...

HOW I'M FEELING RIGHT NOW

BEFORE THE EXPERIMENT, I FEEL ...

You've probably told yourself that before the experiment you're feeling worried, nervous, anxious, etc. That's fine, and perfectly normal.

TAKING STEPS TOWARDS WORRY

As I mentioned, I'm not going to make you walk up to your worry all at once. So for example, if you worry about talking in public, and you feel it's stopping you from taking part in class discussions, we can tackle this worry, one stage at a time. The first stage might be to put your hand up in class if you know the answer to a question the teacher has asked. You'll be feeling nervous, and you might even start to sweat and shake a little, but that's okay.

So now imagine that you answered the question, and even though you felt nervous, nothing terrible happened! The next stage might be to take part in a class discussion and, instead of putting up your hand in response to a question, you volunteer information and opinions. Again, you might feel nervous and sick, but again, nothing terrible happens.

Then we move on to stage three, in which you prepare a two-minute presentation which you deliver in front of the class. This will feel difficult, but you are courageous and it all goes well. Then you might move to stage four, in which you take part in a school play, remembering lines and performing in front of your friends. And if you can do this, you're well on your way to success.

Another example might be that you're worried about taking an exam because you think you will fail and let people down. What do you think would happen if you made one or two small mistakes in an essay? The teacher might point them out, but he or she won't fail you just because of a small mistake or two. And if you take the exam, but don't get the best grade, it really won't be as bad as you'd feared. The people that you thought you'd let down aren't as bothered as you thought they would be. And you won't be either.

THE WORRY LADDER

To start the experiment we're going to put a 'Worry Ladder' against a wall.

We will place our Worry-Goal (i.e. what we would like to achieve by embracing our worry) right at the top of the ladder. For example, let's have a look at Amie's story ...

Amie has a shock of red hair! She also has a lot of freckles on her arms and on her face. Amie's mum says she is a 'natural beauty' but Amie doesn't believe her and is embarrassed about being a 'ginger'. She wears lots of make-up, hats and long-sleeved tops to hide her hair and freckles. When summer comes, she'd love to wear loose, light clothing like all her friends, but she can't. Amie's Thinking Traps include 'Fortune Telling' and 'Worst-Case Scenario'. She believes that if she shows her red hair and the freckles on her arms, people will stare at her and may also make fun of her.

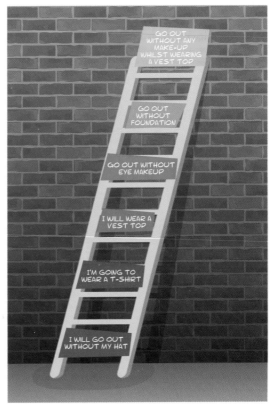

WHAT IS THE EVIDENCE FOR AMIE'S THOUGHT BEING TRUE?

• I do feel very anxious when I think about other people making fun of me.

• Well, that's not a lot of evidence is it?! What's the evidence that Amie's thought is not true?

• Just because I'm anxious it doesn't mean people will make fun of me.

• There are a couple of other people in my year with red hair, so I'm not the only one.

• Most people are more concerned with their own appearance than thinking about what I look like.

• I know that my friends all worry about their appearance too, it's quite normal.

SO, WHAT SHOULD SHE DO?

Amie's Worry-Goal is not to care that she has red hair and freckles, and to wear the clothes all her friends are wearing. So let's put that at the top of her ladder ...

Amie can't get there straight away. She's far too embarrassed, and even the thought of it makes her feel jittery and sick. So, to get her started, let's ask her to take off her hat and see how it feels.

'It was okay,' she said. 'A few people said, "Hello Ginger!" but they were only joking. Most of my friends said what lovely hair I have, and how they'd secretly quite like to have red hair too.'

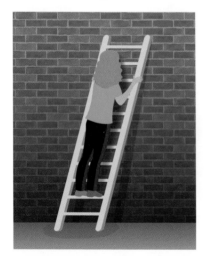

Well done, Amie – take the first step up the ladder! Next, Amie decides to wear a T-shirt, it means everyone will be able to see the freckles on her arms. At first she feels as if everyone is staring at her but then one of her friends points out that she has more freckles than Amie. So she feels okay about herself, and takes another step up the ladder.

Next, she tries on a vest-top and finds this pretty easy after wearing the T-shirt, so she goes up another rung. Now, she is on the last-but-one step to the top. Amie's final step is to go out without wearing all the thick make-up she usually applies to hide her freckles. This feels really hard. Amie hesitates and thinks about quitting, but decides to give it a go.

'It felt so weird at first,' she said. 'People were saying, "you look so different!" and made some positive comments about my new look. At first I wondered if they were saying that I looked ugly, but I looked at their body language and how they actually said it and decided I was reading them wrongly. So I told myself, "They're saying I look good!" and after that, I felt much better about myself. And it doesn't make me feel sick or worried any more.'

After a lot of effort, Amie finally climbed to the top of the ladder and embraced her worry. She'd done it!

So you see, if you approach your worry in stages you'll find it much easier to embrace it when you eventually get there. It won't be anywhere near as scary (in fact, it might not be scary at all now) and you'll feel you've really proved something to yourself.

Now it's your turn! Are you ready?

First, let's write down your experiment. I will show you what Amie wrote before she did hers, and you can fill out the details of your experiment in the blank box below.

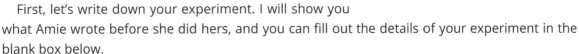

AMIE'S EXPERIMENT

MY EXPERIMENT IS TO ...
Wear the summer clothes I like and not wear as much make up or a hat everywhere.

ON THE ONE HAND ...
The problem is that everyone might laugh at me and make mean comments. People always laugh at 'gingers', don't they?

ON THE OTHER HAND ...
My worry problem is telling me that it's me worrying about it and most people will not even notice or care what I look like! Most people are more concerned with making sure they look good, and don't worry about how other people look.

MY EXPERIMENT, AND THE TWO HANDS TEST

MY EXPERIMENT IS TO ...
_____
_____
_____

ON THE ONE HAND ...
The problem is ...
_____
_____
_____

ON THE OTHER HAND ...
_____
_____
_____
_____

So that was Amie's experiment challenge. In the box above, write down your experiment and fill in your thoughts about the 'One Hand' and the 'Other Hand' theories.

How did you get on? Did it make you feel more comfortable about your own experiment? If so, give it a go now.

Remember – set big goals, but take small steps towards them … !

Okay, so hopefully now you've given your experiment a go. How did you get on? Was it comfortable / uncomfortable? Did it turn out the way your worries told you it might, or did something else happen?

Let's look at Amie's responses to her experiment …

Q: DID THE 'ONE HAND' PREDICTION COME TRUE?

A: No. A few people said, 'Hello Ginger,' but they were being friendly. Most people said I looked good and they liked my new look!

Q: HOW DID YOU FEEL?

A: Anxious at first, and very conscious of my hair, but pleased that people liked it.

Q: IF THE 'OTHER HAND' POSITION IS TRUE IT MEANS YOU HAVE A WORRY-BASED PROBLEM THAT MAKES YOU ANXIOUS. SO, WHAT SHOULD YOU DO NOW?

A: Stop worrying!

Q: WHAT DID YOU LEARN FROM THIS EXPERIMENT?

A: That I need to work on my worry.

Q: IS YOUR WORRY STILL THERE?

A: Yes, because I don't know if people might laugh at me in the future.

Q: HOW CAN YOU EXPERIMENT WITH THIS?

A: By seeing what happens when I wear a vest top and remove my make-up!

Now, fill in the box below with you own experience:

Q: DID THE 'ONE HAND' PREDICTION COME TRUE?

Q: HOW DID YOU FEEL?

Q: IF THE 'OTHER HAND' POSITION IS TRUE AND IT'S A WORRY-BASED PROBLEM THAT MAKES YOU ANXIOUS, WHAT SHOULD YOU DO NOW?

Q: WHAT DID YOU LEARN FROM THIS EXPERIMENT?

Q: IS YOUR WORRY STILL THERE?

Q: WHAT EXPERIMENTS CAN YOU DO NOW TO MOVE YOU UP THE LADDER?

TAKE YOUR TIME

So you've learned how to carry out the experiments. Now you just need to keep doing them and you'll find yourself moving, bit by bit, up the worry ladder. Don't get upset if you have a wobble now and again; this is completely normal. There may well be days when you think, 'Why am I doing this!?' 'Will it ever work!? Will I ever get better!?'

Yes, you will. I know this process works. But it does take time to do the experiments, so try to be patient.

SOME MORE EXPERIMENTS FOR YOU TO TRY

Whatever your worry is, you can always find an experiment to challenge and embrace it. Here are a few of the more common ones, and the ways in which the young people involved have tackled them.

- Sofia was worried about her house catching fire if she left appliances on. So she deliberately left a light on while she was at school.
- Tim worried whether people would like his Facebook post on the charity work he was doing, but he posted it anyway.
- Mistie worried about not making the volleyball team. She thought it would be better not to try, rather than risk the disappointment of not being picked. But she tried out anyway.
- Naomi worried because she only had an old phone. She thought she'd be laughed at if she used it in front of her friends. But she used it anyway.
- Kyle was a good singer and he was asked to sing a solo on stage at school. He worried about people thinking he was nervous, but he did it anyway.
- Chloe was frightened someone would break into her house. So she deliberately left the door unlocked and went for a 20-minute walk.
- Sara always worried about making mistakes, so she purposely made a few spelling errors in her last English essay.

Did anything happen? Did any of their worries come true? Probably not. But suppose they did ...

Let's imagine someone said, 'I can't believe you're still using that crappy old phone' to Naomi. This might have upset Naomi for a moment. But, after that, nothing else bad happened. Naomi felt a bit shaky and sick inside when her friend mentioned her phone. But she knows that she did a brave thing and decided to try another experiment. She decided to get her phone out again the next time she met her friends. And this time, it didn't feel quite so scary. The thing that Naomi had feared had already been said, and this time, no one mentioned it at all.

Remember that it's the worry itself that is causing you problems, not the reality! To a large extent you can't control what happens in the future, but you can control your worries **about** the future by accepting and embracing them.

SHIFTING YOUR ATTENTION

Sometimes you can get caught up worrying about worry and you begin to examine yourself for signs that anxiety is kicking in. This is what we call 'Selective Attention', which means paying very close attention to symptoms or signs that things are 'not okay'. For example, if you hate speaking in public and you have to do it in class, you might notice your heart is racing, you could even imagine you were having a heart attack. So suddenly, you pay a lot more attention to your heart rate.

You might also find that you start to 'scan' your environment for signs of danger. For example, you might interpret someone's body language as a sign of a threat to you. If this is the case, you can try to **shift your attention** away from that particular worry or physical sensation. This is a good tactic if you're feeling anxious because you're about to make a presentation, noticing all your physiological signs of attention, or you feel like you're fixating on worries.

Remember Zak? He tried to avoid his problems – but that kind of 'Safety Behaviour' actually makes the problem worse. Shifting your attention is an entirely different approach. It isn't avoidance; we're actually doing something positive to stop the Worry Wheel spinning.

It also helps to do this if you can't stop the worries or intrusive thoughts popping into your head. (We speak more about intrusive thoughts in the OCD section, but they can happen to anyone with a worry problem.)

Let's set an exercise to help with this. You'll need a quiet room, and an alarm clock (or use the alarm on your phone).

1) Set your alarm for 30 seconds, close your eyes and focus on your worry.

2) When 30 seconds is up, open your eyes, have a look around the space you're in and pick an object.

3) Focus on the object you've chosen for a few seconds and spend a minute describing the object out loud, in as much detail as possible.

4) Now check in with how you feel. Do you feel less anxious now than you did at the start of the exercise when you were asked to focused on your worry? Hopefully you will, because you have actively chosen to shift your attention away from something that is worrying you, and on to something more positive. Remember, the worry hasn't changed at all – but now you're giving it much less attention!

Let's hear from Jake, who tried this exercise …

'I have a birthmark on my face, and I'm always worried that people judge me on that, and not on who I really am. When I tried this exercise at first I found it hard to concentrate on my worry because I'm so used to trying to block it out. But after 30 seconds I

felt anxious and couldn't stop the thoughts about my birthmark snowballing. Then I opened my eyes and looked at my electric guitar. There was loads about it that I'd never really noticed before – just little details, like the shine of the metal of the bridge and where the frets had worn down. Studying it so closely helped me to forget about the anxiety I was feeling, and when I'd finished I didn't feel anywhere near as worried about my birthmark.

Now have another go at this in a different location. You can do it anywhere you like. Say you're on the bus ... Think of your worry, then open your eyes and have a look at all the passengers' shoes. What do you notice about all the colours, shapes and styles? Think it all out in your head and see how this method of shifting attention works.

WHAT IF MY WORRIES COME TRUE? OMG!!!!!

You still might be thinking about your worries coming true, and what will happen if they do. If so, let me help you by showing you three different scenarios:

Remember what we said regarding worries – that they are mostly future-based. In other words, they haven't happened yet, but you worry that THEY WILL happen at some time in the future.

- **Scenario 1:** You don't know what is going to happen in the future and therefore you can't change what eventually happens.
- **Scenario 2:** You know what's going to happen in the future and you still can't change it.
- **Scenario 3:** You know what will happen in the future and you can affect the outcome of it.

Let's apply this to Madelyn's worry:

Madelyn's friend Evie is moving to another city, leaving Madelyn behind. This has really upset Madelyn because Evie's her best friend. She worries that she will never make another best friend again. Like most people who worry, Madelyn's worry falls either into Scenario 1 or Scenario 2 (in this case it's Scenario 2). So if she can't change it – and she can't – then it's a waste of time worrying about it. However, what can she change? Madelyn knows that Evie is moving away, so instead of worrying about that and the outcome, she can spend time getting to know other girls in her school and save up money to visit Evie once she has settled into her new home (Scenario 3).

The point is that we can't change Scenarios 1 and 2, but we can change Scenario 3 – and knowing that we can change it, we're not likely to be as worried about it. Remember, worries trick us into thinking we can do something about them – but we can't! So really, in Scenario 1 and 2 we are worrying about something we have no control over. Think back to the Thinking Traps and the one about 'Mastery of the Universe', in which we believe we can control everything, when in reality there are many things which are totally beyond our control.

By thinking about our worries this way, we can work out whether it's worth wasting energy worrying about something we can't change, or whether this energy could be better used on something we can change. Accepting this might not always be easy or pleasant, and it might seem as though we're 'giving up' – but we're not. In fact, we're acknowledging that life is not perfect, and our feelings are not always going to be comfortable.

To finish this section, let's see how Bella changed the way she thought about her worry ...

Bella worried that she wouldn't do well in her end-of-year exams, which would affect her overall grades. She worried about this having an effect on her chances of going to university. Whenever she thought about university, she started to get anxious. Her worry made it so hard for her to concentrate on her studies that she began to avoid revising altogether. Eventually she decided to see whether there was another interpretation she could tell herself about her worry. She realised that there was not a 100 per cent guarantee that she would get the grades she wanted, and that there was no point worrying because it wouldn't help. She decided to look at the idea that while going to university would be her dream, there were other things she could do if she didn't get the grades.

But even so, she still worried!

Bella took small steps to face her worry, breaking it down and doing a little bit at a time. Instead of plunging into her revision straight away, and feeling panicky about it, she lay on her bed and listened to her favourite song. On the first night she did ten minutes of revision, then put it away. On the second night, she listened to her favourite song, and did 20 minutes' work. And every night after that, she did ten minutes' more work (once she'd listened to her favourite song). Soon, she was doing an hour a night. Bella still worried a little bit about the exam, but the strategy to beat the worry by organising her revision time worked, and finally she passed the exam and made it to university!

Bella's One Hand interpretation of her thought was that she wouldn't do well in her exams and then she wouldn't get the grades she needed to go to uni. As a result she worried that her life would be ruined. But on the Other Hand, Bella reasoned that there are no guarantees in life – and if she really didn't get the grades she wanted, then she would cope. She could try again, or find other things to do instead.

TESTING IT ALL OUT | 165

REASSURANCE

Before we leave this chapter, let's have a look at the idea of **Reassurance**. I can almost guarantee that if you've tried to tell someone about your worries and anxieties, they've probably replied, 'Don't worry – everything will be okay!' And maybe you've gone away thinking, 'Well, they say it will be okay, so maybe it will be okay?' Now you've got the reassurance you think you needed until ... your worries, doubts and anxieties creep in again, and then you need to seek even more reassurance.

One problem with reassurance is that it feeds anxiety. For example, you might be like Adam, and have an uncomfortable thought about hurting another person. What do you do with that thought? If you attach importance to it, you will probably start Googling to see if you're a psychopath or a serial killer. As we know, there is a lot of misinformation on the internet and you might read something that really doesn't help you at all! You might also seek reassurance that bad things won't happen, by asking repeated questions of yourself and others ('Am I ill?' 'Am I mad?' 'Did I switch the electricity off?' 'Did I close the door properly?' 'Do I really look like this?' 'Do other people like me?' etc.)

The other problems with reassurance are that it reinforces the fear that something is bad or wrong. Second, your anxiety problem is very clever and reassurance will never ever be enough – it will always need more and more reassurance. Third, especially on the internet, you can almost always find something that confirms your fears, however wrong it is, which will only make you feel worse.

So although it is tempting, please try not to rely on reassurance. Your friends and family mean well, but, if you practise the challenges and experiments we've talked about above, you won't need their reassurance. You already have the power to make yourself feel better.

Let's have a look at a quick exercise in seeking reassurance. If you seek reassurance, think about the ways you do it. Then think about how you might stop it. Here's an example. If it helps, fill in the rest of the box with your own reassurance-seeking and ways to stop it.

> **HOW I SEEK REASSURANCE**
> (Example)
> **I Google to see if I'm going mad**
>
> **HOW I CAN STOP SEEKING REASSURANCE**
> **Turn off my laptop or phone and do something else instead!**

Finally, do remember to keep trying your experiments. The more you repeat them, the more your worries and anxiety will lessen, and the more successful you will be. There will be times when you feel uncomfortable, but keep going! And remember to be kind to yourself at all times.

CHAPTER SUMMARY

• We carry out experiments to test out theories and ideas – not to prove we are right!

• Before you carry out your experiments, you may be feeling anxious, worried and nervous. That's completely normal, so go forward with courage.

• Set big goals, but take small steps towards them.

• Selective attention describes how we can get caught up worrying about worry – paying attention to the symptoms and signs that tell us we are not okay. But we've seen how we can shift attention away from your worries without pushing them away so that they return.

• What if your worries come true? Well, worrying about them beforehand won't change that! And if they do come true, the results are usually not as bad as you think.

• We can tell ourselves **a different story** about our worries too – this makes it easier to embrace them.

• Try not to reassure yourself, or allow others to reassure you, about your worries. Carrying out the experiment to tackle your worries is a much better plan!

• It's important to keep repeating experiments and pushing further. Feeling uncomfortable is good – it means that you are still challenging yourself. That's how you'll make the most progress.

Chapter 21

CONTROL

The final part of our recovery approach is **CONTROL**. Control is our way of describing how we manage our worries and anxieties after we've understood how to Accept and Embrace them.

CONTROL, NOT FIGHT

You might not be surprised to hear that our version of 'Control' isn't quite like the one you'd expect.

It's not about shouting, 'I AM IN CONTROL!!'

It's not about a 'fight' or a 'battle' with worry or anxiety.

In fact, 'Control' is not about control at all. It's quite the opposite ...

I AM IN CONTROL!

What I'm asking you to do is control your anxiety and worry by allowing it in.

That's right. Accepting and embracing your anxiety and worry – seeing it for what it is – is the key to controlling it. You do not need to do anything big or dramatic or shouty. Worries are just thoughts (including images, doubts, urges and sensations), and you can go forward to meet those worries face-to-face.

Every time you do this, **it puts you in control**. Every time you embrace your worries, the level of your anxiety drops.

Adam's way of controlling his anxiety and worry is to say 'Bring it on!' Quite often, he seeks out a situation which he knows has the potential to make him anxious, and he tests himself against it. He embraces it, sits with it and even welcomes it in – because each time he does this, he feels that little bit better.

UPS AND DOWNS, AND HOW TO DEAL WITH THEM

That said, there will be days when you feel bad. There may be times when you feel like nothing is working out. This feeling can be very strong in the recovery stage. You're at a point where you feel you're making great progress and then suddenly ...

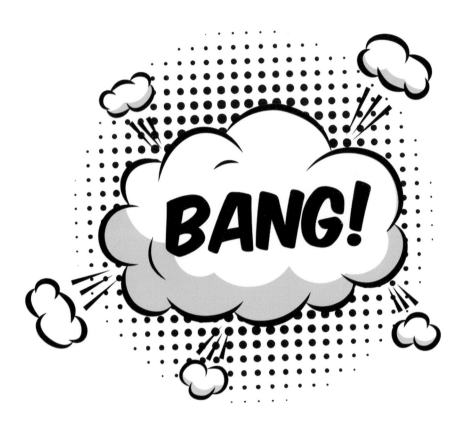

You're down in the dumps and feeling anxious again.

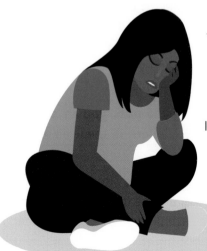

That is completely normal. And the best way to deal with it? You guessed it ... you need to accept and embrace it.

Accept that you will have bad days, and let the feelings sit with you. They will pass. All feelings eventually change, and all strong feelings eventually reduce. This is what we call 'The Impermanence of Emotions', which is a wordy way of saying that nothing lasts forever. You might not believe it when you're experiencing them, but strong or intense feelings do eventually decrease.

Below is a graph to explain what I mean:

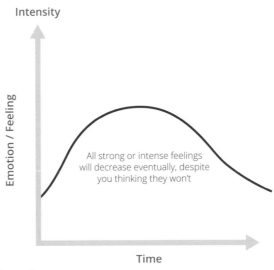

Figure 5: *Impermanence of emotions.*

And as you sit with these feelings, take a **'be kind to yourself'** approach – read a book, listen to music, play a computer game, watch a DVD, hang out with your friends. These aren't ways of avoiding the feelings you're having. They're just **helpful distractions**, ways of passing the time while you let the feelings of worry and anxiety wash over you. Acknowledge the feeling but choose to do something distracting to be kind to yourself, and allow the feeling to naturally reduce in intensity.

It is okay not to feel okay, because you are a human, and that is part of being human.

When you use helpful distractions, you will notice that the strong feelings you're having will reduce in intensity. Even when your emotions and feelings are at their peak, helpful distractions will bring them down. Below is a graph which shows this.

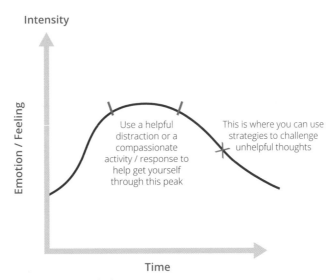

Figure 6: *How to manage strong emotions / feelings.*

As time goes on, and you're accepting and embracing your anxiety and being kind to yourself, you will notice the anxiety lessening. Now you're making progress. Your mood is brighter and you feel there are better times ahead.

BUT!

Quite often it's at this point that a bad day can really bring you down again. You've started to feel much better and suddenly you're back in that scary space again. You might think, 'Oh, this hasn't worked' or 'It's all been a waste of time', but please remember, this is normal. Recovering from an anxiety-based, or obsessional illness is like recovering from any illness; some days you'll feel great, others you won't. If you're into sports, you'll know that a sports injury takes time to heal properly. And it's exactly the same with your mind. You might feel irritated and frustrated. You might even feel despair, but you should remember that just as a sprained ankle doesn't go on forever, neither does a spell of anxiety or OCD. You might feel all 'Worst-Case Scenario' but if you didn't have days when you felt up and down, you wouldn't be making progress. Below is a Recovery Graph to show you what I mean:

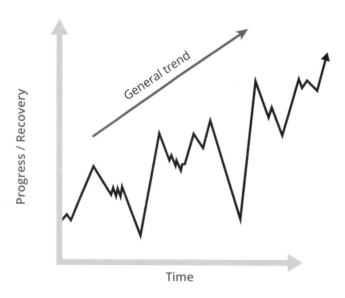

Figure 7: *Progress and recovery over time.*

Yes, it does look pretty crazy, and a bit 'up and down'. But that's just how it will be for a while. The important thing is that you are going in the right direction – you are heading towards recovery.

RELAXATION

An important part of the recovery stage is finding time for relaxation. This isn't always easy, as you have so many things going on in your life right now, but it's very beneficial just to take a step back, breathe deeply and learn to relax.

There are many great ways to relax, using different techniques that you can find in books and on the net. Below is one of the best for worry and anxiety.

1) Find a quiet space in your house and take a few moments to lie down and stretch out.

2) Then, with your eyes closed, tense every muscle in your body, starting from your toes, up through your stomach, from your fingertips up your arms and into your neck and jaw.

3) Once everything is tense, take a deep breath and begin to relax each muscle, one at a time. Again, start with your feet ... uncurl your toes, and allow this sensation to drift up your legs, thighs, buttocks and glutes.

4) Relax your stomach, then your fingers and arms and finally your neck and face.

5) When you are fully relaxed, take time to focus on a really good memory; a holiday, a day out with friends or something that went really well at school.

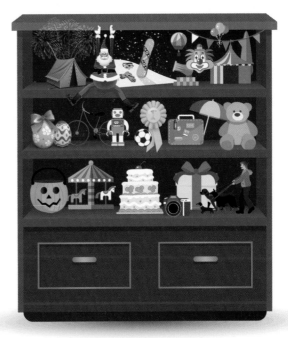

6) Try to remember all the details: what the weather was like, what you were wearing, what your friends said, what you ate and drank – all the things that made the day so pleasurable.

7) When you've explored this, store it away in your memory where you can easily access it next time you feel worried or anxious.

MINDFULNESS

You might have heard about a technique called 'mindfulness', which is a way of allowing thoughts or feelings to float around our heads without judging them or giving them unnecessary attention. Mindfulness is a very useful way of managing the times you feel worried or anxious. Here's a useful mindfulness exercise for you to try.

1) Close your eyes and pretend you're on a beach, or by a lake, or in a grassy meadow.

2) When you 'see' your worries coming along in your mind, imagine turning them into clouds and watch them float by, and away.

3) You don't have to give them any importance, or pay any more attention to them than they deserve ...

4) Just let them drift off ...

Relaxation doesn't have to involve closing your eyes or lying down. It can be doing something peaceful that you enjoy. Many people find sport or cookery relaxing. Others read, play games, or listen to music. One of my clients, Sabrina, used to paint her nails as a way of relaxation. And it worked!

If you think that mindfulness will be a good tactic for you, there are lots of good apps and downloads you can investigate to will help you.

GET UP AND GO!

People relax in all sorts of different ways. It can involve sports and activities that require high levels of fitness and concentration. Swimming, running, go-karting, horse-riding, and most other active sports burn nervous energy and this really helps recovery from worry and anxiety.

If worry and anxiety have caused you to give up a sport or a pastime that you used to enjoy, the recovery stage is the time to get back into that activity. It will give you a real energy boost and a sense of achievement. Remember – these activities aren't ways of avoiding feelings of worry and anxiety. If they do come along, you need to pay attention to them in the way we've shown you. Sports, pastimes and other activities are 'helpful distractions'.

Let's see what happened when Simon used sport to assist his recovery ...

'I found school quite challenging because I was pretty average in most things and the pressure was on to get better grades. I found that I was worrying about exams to the point where I couldn't face revising.

The one thing I'm good at, though, is sport, mainly basketball. So if I knew I had to sit through a period of revision, I'd do 15 minutes' revision and then, as a reward, I'd shoot hoops for 10 minutes. Then I'd do 20 minutes' revision and shoot hoops for 15 minutes. I found that my concentration improved massively, and my shooting technique really went up too! So it was win-win all round.'

Being more active can also help you to improve your sleep patterns ...

ARE YOU GETTING ENOUGH SLEEP?

You've probably found that the more anxious you are, the harder it is to get good quality sleep. And the less sleep you get, the more likely it is that you will suffer with anxiety. It's a vicious cycle.

There's no doubt about it, sleep is one of the most important things you can do to help your recovery from anxiety and OCD. It gives you the energy and the focus you need to deal with your anxiety in a positive way.

Think about how you feel after missing one night's sleep ... a bit cranky, short on concentration? Now imagine how you'd feel if you had a whole week of interrupted sleep. Or a month ... Some people with severe OCD and anxiety never get a proper night's sleep. They lie awake night after night, thinking over their worries and their strategies to try and make things better.

So what do you do to break the cycle and get your sleep back on track?

HERE ARE SOME IDEAS:

- Whatever you do, don't lie there worrying. If you're not asleep within 20 minutes, get out of bed and go and do something else. Read a book. Listen to some quiet music, and best of all, practise shifting your attention on to other things. Don't watch TV or use your phone or other electronic devices though. This will only make you more alert when you need your body to relax and get ready for sleep.

- When you can't sleep, you really do need to get out of bed. It's important to try and associate bed with sleep and comfort, not anxiety. (Don't panic. The sleep cycle is like a wave. At some points the body feels more ready for sleep than others. You will find yourself getting tired again.)

- If your worries just won't let you sleep, write them down. That way you know you won't forget them. You can worry about them again in the morning. But, after a night of uninterrupted rest, many people find that their worries don't seem quite so urgent in the morning.

- If you need to complete rituals before you go to bed, then try to start on them earlier. At least that way, you'll have a better chance of getting a bit more sleep.

- You don't have to try and sleep more than necessary. Up to the age of 17, you probably need about nine hours' sleep a night. But as you get older this'll drop down. Try and get into a regular routine, so that you're in bed, ready to sleep by 10 or 11pm – and aim to get up at the same time each morning.

- Don't eat big meals within the two or three hours before you go to bed if possible – and lay off the fizzy drinks, energy drinks – and alcohol!

- It's tempting to nap in the day if you feel tired, but don't. It'll only interfere with your night-time sleep routine and make it harder to develop lasting sleep patterns.

- Your body craves darkness – it helps to prepare it for sleep. So make sure your room is as dark as possible. If there is a lot of streetlight outside, try a blackout blind. Remember – no phone, tablet, or TV 30 minutes before bed.

- Aim to go to bed at the same time every night. It helps your body get ready for sleep.

Developing a sleep routine can feel like hard work to begin with – but do stick with it. It really is worth it. I promise you'll feel so much better when you get used to having a proper night's sleep every night.

In the box below, have a think about writing down some ways you would find helpful to relax, and list some new ones that you would like to try.

CHAPTER SUMMARY

- 'Control' is not about control at all. In fact, it's the opposite. You control your anxiety and worry by allowing it in.

- There will be times you feel bad, or uncomfortable, or weird. That's fine, because those things are normal, and accepting and embracing these feelings is the best way to deal with them.

- Having ups and downs is a sign you're making progress, so don't panic.

- Nothing lasts forever, and that includes strong feelings and emotions.

- Take a 'Be Kind to Yourself' approach and remember that …

- It is okay not to feel okay, because you are a human, and that is part of being human.

- Relaxation is a vital part of recovery. Relaxing can be a quiet or an energetic experience – it's up to you!

- Mindfulness is a very useful way of managing the times you feel worried or anxious.

- Having a good sleep routine is an essential component in helping you address your anxiety and OCD.

- Relaxation, mindfulness and activities you enjoy are great ways of dealing with worry and anxiety.

Chapter 22

Obsessive Compulsive Disorder

Now we're going to look a little more closely at OCD, but before we do, can I check that you've read the Anxiety and Worry chapters? Pretty much everything that's written in those chapters applies to anyone who thinks they might have Obsessive-Compulsive Disorder (OCD).

These days, we hear a lot about people being 'a bit OCD' or having 'a touch of OCD'. Some kids – and adults! – tease each other about it. But generally, it doesn't mean anything more than pointing out that we all have funny little ways or habits. For example, a friend of mine feels uncomfortable at night if his wardrobe door is open and he has to shut the door before he gets into bed. The wardrobe door being open (or not) won't make any **real** difference to how he actually sleeps, but the uncomfortable feeling is there so he still shuts the door.

Doing this doesn't make any major difference to his life, and it doesn't upset him in a big way. It's just a silly routine based on a superstition which he could easily break if he wanted to. However, if he started to worry about all doors, drawers and cupboards being open right through the house, and spent 30 minutes or so checking each room (and waking other people up!) then we'd say he had a problem.

SO WHAT IS OCD?

Real OCD is an **obsessional problem that can be about anything, causing us to feel anxious, depressed, disgusted, ashamed and guilty**. In brief, OCD is when people have intrusions that are very upsetting, which they *interpret* to be very threatening. Of course this makes people feel worried, anxious and fearful, so that they naturally want to minimise or *reduce the threat* and stop themselves having these pesky intrusive thoughts at all!

These intrusions can include unpleasant thoughts images, doubts, or sensations along with the 'compulsive' urge to get rid of them or 'neutralise' them (i.e. make them safe or undo the intrusion) in some way. People with OCD avoid situations, or 'triggers', that involve their obsessions, they carry out repetitive behaviours, rituals or safety behaviours (checking, counting, washing, cleaning, etc.) and seek reassurance from others that 'everything is okay' and that what they fear happening won't actually happen.

This sounds a lot like worry, but it's not the same ...

Worry might dominate your life, but it doesn't give you an obsessive urge to carry out rituals and complicated habits to try and make the anxiety go away. Think back to Adam's story and how he had to do everything four times – from turning on and off the bath taps to kicking the football – until everything felt 'just right' – that moment when you decide that a compulsion can stop because it feels 'just right'. For example, if your compulsion is washing your hands, only you will know when it feels 'just right' to stop. This could last for any length of time, from a few minutes up to several hours. There is no fixed point because the aim is to get it 'just right'. You're trying to get relief but you're not basing this on anything real. Your level for 'just right' may change constantly depending on how you feel that day. It is a subjective and unscientific way of deciding when to stop.

LET'S FIND OUT MORE ABOUT HOW YOU'RE FEELING ...

While some obsessions are more common than others, OCD can be about absolutely anything. So let me ask you some questions which you can answer in the boxes below:

ARE YOU HAVING THOUGHTS, DOUBTS, IMAGES, URGES OR SENSATIONS THAT ARE DISTRESSING AND UNWANTED?

Yes / no

IF 'YES', WHAT ARE THEY ABOUT?

(It can be hard to admit these, especially if you find them very uncomfortable but please remember that everyone has strange / unpleasant / weird thoughts from time to time!)

_____

_____

_____

_____

_____

_____

ARE THESE THOUGHTS CAUSING YOU ANXIETY OR UPSET OR SOME FORM OF DISTRESS?

Yes / no

IF 'YES', WHAT ARE YOU DOING IN RESPONSE TO THEM? (WRITE DOWN ANY COMPULSIONS, RITUALS OR 'SAFETY BEHAVIOURS' INCLUDING THINGS YOU MAY BE AVOIDING.)

_____

_____

_____

_____

_____

IT'S ALL MY FAULT!

If you have OCD, you interpret your intrusive thought as being **'Worst-Case Scenario'** (see page 136) and feel compelled to carry out rituals because you feel that you have a responsibility to stop this bad thing from happening. This is a thinking trap we call 'Me To The Rescue'! To ensure it doesn't happen, you also might carry out lots of different safety behaviours and also try and prevent yourself having more intrusions.

OCD can make you feel responsible for everything. The **'Me to the Rescue'** thinking trap wants to take over your life so you feel that everything that happens – or might happen – is your fault ('Blame and Shame'). It makes you feel that things have the potential for a terrible ending ('Worst-Case Scenario') and it is your fault for not stopping it from happening. Here's a quick guide to some of the commonest types of OCD worries:

- Contamination worries. A compulsive need to clean and wash to protect against contamination which may cause illness or death to yourself or a loved one, or make you feel unclean or dirty in some way.

- Checking worries. A compulsion to check and re-check to protect against the fear of damage, leaks, fires etc. Among the commonest checks are stoves, hobs and cookers, door locks, lights, taps, and appliances. Checks may also include repeatedly texting people to check they're alright, checking driving routes for fear of causing an accident.

- Strange sexual thoughts. A fear that ranges from checking one's own sexuality (e.g. being homosexual or being attracted to family members) to worrying about causing sexual harm to children or others (e.g. being a paedophile).

- A person with religious worries may fear that they will say something blasphemous in a religious place, or that they are doing something sinful. They may fear they have broken religious thoughts, had inappropriate sexual thoughts about God and saints, or fear that their sins will never be forgiven, meaning they will go to hell.

- People who worry about bodily functions become hyper-aware of their breathing, swallowing, or blinking. They may fixate on specific parts and functions of their body.

- The compulsion of having to have everything ordered or symmetrical helps people to feel that they can prevent some harm from occurring. Typical examples are making sure pictures are straight, having food items, books or clothing neatly arranged and facing the same way etc.

- Causing harm in some way to others, or causing something else terrible to happen, either deliberately, or by accident, for example not moving a stone you see in the road, which someone on a bike later hits and is killed or injured. (Of course, that is just one example of OCD behaviour.)

All these things 'might' happen. But are you sure they're 100 per cent guaranteed to be totally your fault all the time?

That depends on the meaning we attach to the intrusions. So, for example, if you have an intrusive thought about hurting your little brother or sister, the meaning you attach to it might be something like: 'Oh no, I've had a terrible thought about hurting them. This must mean that I could be a murderer! And I should stay away from them because I'm a danger to children.'

A THOUGHT IN COURT

Let's put one of these thoughts to the test … I'm going to use a really common one – the worry that you might catch germs from something or someone. If you've ever been in a confined space full of people (like a bus or a train or a Tube) or you've sat next to someone at the cinema who is sneezing and blowing their nose, you'll definitely understand this thought!

So let's put this thought on trial, using the **One Hand / Other Hand** method we've already used in the past few chapters.

On the **One Hand** you might think: 'Oh no! The person next to me has sneezed! I'm definitely going to catch germs now, and I might pass them on to members of my family who will fall ill. If my granddad gets it, it could make his chest even worse … he might die! So I'd better get off the bus now, even though I'm still a mile from home, and find the nearest public toilet where I can wash my hands. And then, when I get home, I'll shower and wash, and shower again until I've got all these germs off me and I feel 'right' again!'

On the **Other Hand** you might think: 'Oh no! The person next to me has sneezed. I might get a cold now. But there again, I could get a cold from anyone, and thinking about it, three kids in my class have already got colds, so I might catch it from them. I could move seats but the bus is packed and I'm a mile from home. So I might as well sit here until my stop comes up, and I can get some fresh air then.'

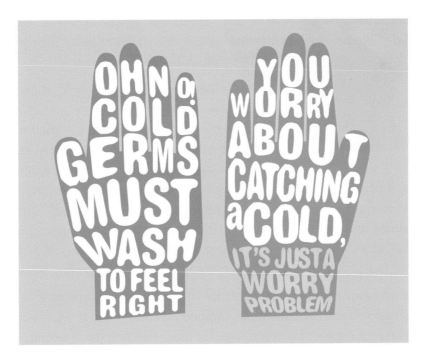

So you see – the 'One Hand' version attaches a **catastrophic (Gloom and Dooming Scenario) meaning** to the thought of germs, making it feel very real and dangerous. You feel **100 per cent responsible (Me To The Rescue)** for the possible outcome, and to stop that thought you carry out a compulsion – you get away from the bus, then wash and shower – in order to feel safe.

The 'Other Hand' point of view also finds the idea of catching germs uncomfortable, but then realises that colds can be caught from anyone, anywhere. The bus is packed and it's a mile from home, so you just accept the situation and treat the thought as sensibly as you can.

In short, with OCD it's NOT the thought that counts – it's the importance and meaning we give to it, and what we do to make ourselves feel better.

Here's an example:

Josh started to worry about getting things right, especially in school. Thoughts about doing things wrong started to crowd his mind. He worried about answering incorrectly in class. He worried about getting into trouble. He worried about not bringing the right bit of kit for PE. He worried that he would fail his exams, and the rest of his life would be ruined. Josh worried a lot, about a lot of things ... and to ease his worries, he developed a ritual. As he walked to school, Josh looked at all the street names and decided that the last one would look at before he went into school should begin with an 'A' – which was the grade he wanted to get in his exams! This was okay for a while, but eventually Josh had to look out for more and more road names beginning with 'A' so that he would feel 'right'. This made him late for school several times, and it got him into trouble (something he really worried about). But he was unable to stop, because if he didn't, the feeling of being 'wrong' would drag him down, deeper and deeper ...

Reading this, you might think: 'That doesn't make any sense! How can a road name influence what grade someone will get in their exam?!' Josh has fallen into a thinking trap. So, to him, it made perfect sense. The meaning he attached to his intrusive thought ('I will fail my exams') was that if he got his checking behaviour wrong he would never feel okay again and would mess up in school. So he had to make sure he got his checking ritual right to feel okay all the time. That's what's strange about OCD – the rituals and behaviours you get caught up in might seem strange to other people, but to you they are a lifeline. They're a way of protecting yourself against the 'dangerous' thoughts and really uncomfortable feelings you feel occupy your mind.

Josh had to do whatever it took to 'feel right'. He was trying to defend himself against thoughts that made him uncomfortable. But his rituals trapped him into doing the same things time after time. That mean he couldn't ever try new things, for fear of getting them wrong.

We already know that the **importance** we give to a thought is crucial to the way it affects us.

Let's have a look at Maisie's story:

Maisie worried that something bad would happen to her family. She loved them, and wanted to keep them from harm. She knew about fires and floods, and the thought of something bad happening disturbed her so much that, last thing at night, when everyone had gone to bed, she took responsibility for checking all the electrical appliances, the gas and water taps. It could take almost two hours on some nights before Maisie felt 'safe' and 'just right'. It meant that she was tired in the morning, and also that her parents were cross with her for wandering around the house late at night. The result was that Maisie started to fall behind at school, was too tired to hang out with her friends, and kept getting into arguments with her mum and dad.

Maisie's intrusive thoughts centred around her family coming to harm. She had fallen into the 'me to the rescue' thinking trap so that she felt it was her responsibility to keep them safe by checking electrical appliances and taps. She also experienced 'gloom and dooming' so that she thought there would be a fire or a flood if she didn't check. Maisie loves her family and didn't want anything bad to happen to them, but her behaviours caused arguments with her parents and created an unhappy situation at home. How ironic!

But what would have happened if she'd put her thought 'on trial' using our **'Two Hands Theory'**?

On the One Hand, her OCD was telling her that she needed to make everything 'safe' so that nothing bad happened to her family or it would be all her fault if something did happen.

BUT ...

On the Other Hand, she might have understood that she couldn't be **responsible** for her whole family's safety, all the time. That would be impossible! And the real problem was her worrying about keeping everyone safe.

So if Maisie had been realistic about her thought, she'd understand that while she can take some responsibility for safety at home (it is a good idea to turn off the cooker if it's been left on accidentally!) she isn't the only one who should do this. Realistically, Maisie doesn't need to check things all the time as it is **unlikely** that anything bad will happen.

YOU ARE NOT ALONE

REMEMBER: It's really important for you to understand that we **all** have odd / silly / weird / uncomfortable thoughts, urges, images, sensations, and doubts. Every single one of us does – kids, adults, old people – every single day. It's part of being human, and it's completely normal. Our problems with OCD begin when we take these thoughts too seriously, making them feel 'important', and try to push them away or reduce their importance with routines, rituals or behaviour that make us feel 'safe in some way', but which get in the way of our life.

What kind of things can become obsessive thoughts? Well, if we listed them all we'd need dozens of pages! **Some of the more common ones include:**

- Worries about the future
- Worries about catching a disease, or giving a disease to others
- Worries about harming people
- Worries about dirt, mess, bodily fluids, and vomit
- Worries about health
- Worries about 'strange' or uncomfortable thoughts
- Worries that you might be 'mad'
- Worries about your sexuality
- Worries about strange or unusual sexual behaviour
- Worries about causing damage or destruction
- Worries about not fitting in
- Worries about not 'feeling right'
- Worries about religion

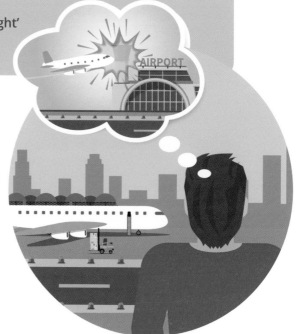

And so on ... There are just too many to list. And the ways we behave in order to make ourselves feel 'safe' or 'just right' are just as long. **Some of the more common ones are:**

- Counting
- Washing / showering
- Checking
- Googling things on the internet
- Putting things in order
- Handwashing
- Mental compulsions (for example, trying to swap a 'bad' thought for a 'good' one, counting, repeating specific phrases)
- Avoiding situations, people or places
- Seeking reassurance from friends or family members and the internet that the worst-case thinking won't happen and you're okay

Please remember – everyone has worries, and everyone has strange, silly or weird thoughts. And occasionally, we do things to try and make these thoughts 'safe'. One very common example is the superstition about walking under ladders. Some people attach a worst-case thought that makes them believe they'll have bad luck if they walk under the ladder. So walking around the ladder is their way of 'protecting' themselves from bad luck.

HOW BIG AN IMPACT DOES YOUR OCD HAVE ON YOUR LIFE?

It is only when your OCD is **significantly interfering in your life** that you have a problem. For example, if Colin switches the hall light off before he leaves for college and checks it again before he closes the door, he is carrying out a ritual but it isn't significantly interfering in his life. However, if Colin walks ten yards down the street, then goes back to check the light switch (and does this several times, making him consistently late for college) the ritual is causing significant interference in his life.

Have a look at the questionnaire below and put a circle round each answer. At the end, add up the scores for choosing 'No', 'A bit', and 'A lot' and see which comes out on top …

QUESTION	SCORE 0	SCORE 1	SCORE 2
Does your mind often make you do things (checking, touching or counting) even though you don't have to?	No	A bit	A lot
Do you feel you have to keep your hands clean?	No	A bit	A lot
Do you have to do a number of things over and over again to get them right?	No	A bit	A lot
Do you have trouble finishing schoolwork or chores because you have to do something over and over?	No	A bit	A lot
Do you worry a lot if you've done something not exactly the way you like it?	No	A bit	A lot

If you answered 'A lot' to any of these questions, please answer the next questions as well.

QUESTION	SCORE 0	SCORE 1	SCORE 2
Do these things interfere with your life in any way?	No	A bit	A lot
How do these things interfere in your life? (write in the space below)			
Do you try to stop them	No	A bit	A lot
How do you try to stop them? (write in the space below)			
Do you try to 'undo' the thoughts or images that are bothering you?	No	A bit	A lot
Do you avoid things because of these thoughts?	No	A bit	A lot
How do these thoughts make you feel?	No	A bit	A lot[3]

Okay – we've established that you're doing something (or even a few things) regularly to try to ensure the doom and gloom meaning doesn't come true, or to prevent having more thoughts like that – and it is interfering in your life. But how? It's worth having a quick look at this, because understanding how your life is being affected by OCD will make you even more determined to get hold of it and shout 'STOP!' right in its face!

Earlier, I told you about Maisie, who was so worried about a fire or flood in her home that she spent up to two hours every night checking the house to make sure she felt 'safe' and 'just right'. That made her really tired every morning and had a big impact on her school work. (And that made her mum and dad cross with her too.)

Adam's story is similar. He was worried that something would happen to his mum after she dropped him off at school. One day he looked up at a cloud and thought that if no one else saw it apart from him, something bad would definitely happen to his mum. After this, he spent a long time trying to force his friends to look at clouds, or else he tried to avoid looking at clouds altogether. This made life very difficult for Adam, because he felt worried and anxious every time he went outside.

Adam's intrusive thought centred around something happening to his mum, and that meant he had to do something to keep her safe. His behaviour involved the appearance of clouds, and trying to force others to see them. So although Adam loved his mum and didn't want anything bad to happen to her, his worries took over and made him stop doing the things he really enjoyed.

IS IT YOUR RESPONSIBILITY?

Do you remember the 'me to the rescue' thinking trap? It made Adam and Maisie take on complete responsibility for making sure the things they worried about didn't happen to their family. But was it really their responsibility?

Let me tell you about Abbie:

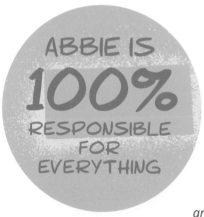

Abbie is her school's top IT student. She is very good at programming, and she is seen as someone with a bright future in IT. But because Abbie knows so much about computers, she knows that sometimes things can go wrong with them – and that worries her a lot. Abbie was asked to be the monitor in the computer room, which meant keeping an eye on them and letting the staff know if there was a problem with the equipment. Quite soon, Abbie feels responsible for all the computers in her school's IT department. She needs to make sure that all the software is updated and anti-virus protected. She needs to make sure that her fellow students are not accessing websites they shouldn't. She also needs to make sure that every computer is properly logged off and powered down at the end of each day. Abbie can hardly sleep at night for thinking that something might happen to the school's computers – and maybe to the school itself – because she hasn't checked, double-checked and triple-checked them. Her constant checking and re-checking drives her fellow-students mad, and often, Abbie is too tired to concentrate on her work.

Is Abbie right to take on 100 per cent responsibility for the school computer room? Well, let's try our On the One Hand and On the Other Hand test and see:

On the **One Hand**, Abbie is 100 per cent responsible for making sure nothing bad happens to the computers.

What is Abbie doing to make sure that nothing bad happens, and what else might she do?

- She checks and re-checks the computers regularly.
- She seeks reassurance from staff that nothing has happened to the computers.
- She might stay late, or comes to school early, to make sure nothing has happened.
- What is the evidence for this position being true?
- Abbie's feelings of responsibility are so strong that only she can protect the department against something going terribly wrong.

On the **Other Hand**, Abbie worries she is responsible for making sure nothing bad happens with the computers, but there are plenty of other people who are responsible too. It is a problem of her worrying about, and not trusting others to make sure they also do their job.

If this position is true, what does Abbie need to do?

Abbie needs to recognise that her problem is around the worry itself, and that many other people have responsibility for the computer department.

What is the evidence for this position being true?

- There are plenty of other people responsible for the computers' safety.
- No one else seems as worried as I am about the computers.
- I feel anxious when I have this thought, which suggests a problem.
- Just because I have these thoughts, it doesn't mean they will come true.
- Everyone has strange or unpleasant or worrying thoughts now and again.

Based on the evidence, which position do you think is more likely to be true? And who is *actually* responsible for the school's computers? As a top IT student trusted by her teachers, Abbie might have a bit of responsibility. But Abbie's classmates also share some of the responsibility. The IT teacher has more responsibility. And the caretaker has even more responsibility. And then there is the company who made the computers. And the internet service provider. And the company who installed the fire alarms.

So when we look at it **on the Other Hand**, we can see that lots of people and organisations have some share of the responsibility.

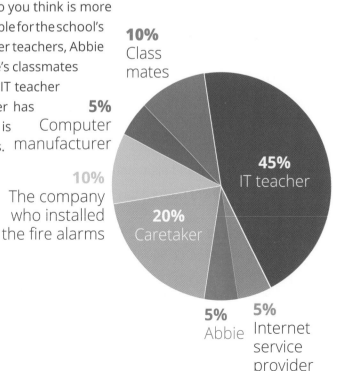

10% Class mates

5% Computer manufacturer

10% The company who installed the fire alarms

20% Caretaker

45% IT teacher

5% Abbie

5% Internet service provider

WHAT ARE MY COMPULSIONS ASKING ME TO DO?

Abbie's compulsions had a massive impact on her daily life. They affected her sleep and her school work. They made life very hard for her.

How are your compulsions interfering in *your* life?

In the box below, write some or all of the habits that you do most, and can't seem to stop. Then answer the rest of the questions ...

MY COMPULSIONS ARE ...

_____

_____

_____

_____

_____

_____

_____

_____

_____

DO YOU CARRY THEM OUT

A) An hour a day?

B) Two hours a day?

C) Between three and eight hours a day?

D) More than eight hours a day?

HOW MUCH IS YOUR LIFE AFFECTED BY THEM
(e.g: your school work, socialising time, hobbies, family, etc.)

A) Not at all

B) Sometimes

C) A lot

D) Always

IF YOUR COMPULSIONS ARE AFFECTING YOUR LIFE A LOT, DESCRIBE HOW ...

_____

_____

_____

_____

_____

_____

_____

_____

_____

_____

_____

IF YOU WERE ABLE TO STOP YOUR COMPULSIONS, OR YOU WERE PREVENTED FROM DOING THEM, HOW WOULD YOU FEEL?

A) Happy?   **E)** Upset?

B) Scared?   **F)** Anxious?

C) Nervous?   **G)** Relieved?

D) Guilty?   **H)** A combination of all the above?

So maybe now you can see how your life is being affected by your compulsions? You may feel a combination of these feelings, but hopefully you will also feel some relief. Although you might worry about what will happen in your life after OCD, I hope you can see that it will likely hold many positives! That makes your journey to recovery so much easier.

THE REVOLVING DOOR OF WORRY

At the moment you are still worrying though, and doing things to try to stop those worries. It probably feels like a trap – a bit like being in one of those revolving doors, only in this revolving door, you can't seem to find the exit! Essentially, that's how OCD works. Your obsessions cause the anxiety – and this pushes you to carry out your compulsions until you feel less anxious, 'safe' or 'just right'. But then, the thought enters your head again, and sets you off again, going round and round, just like being in a never-ending revolving door.

Here's a diagram of how that looks ...

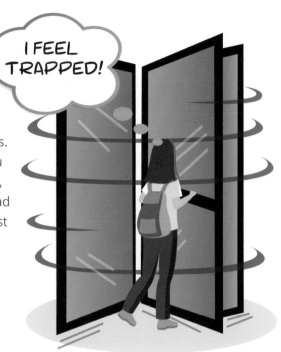

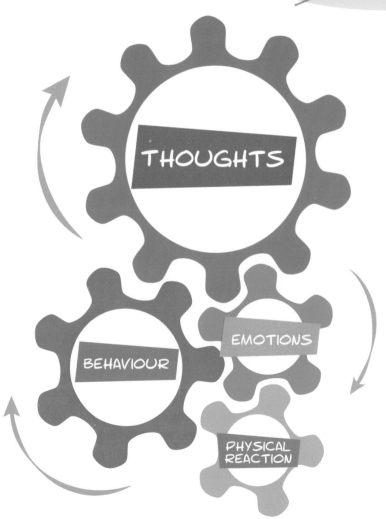

If we think back to Adam's story for a moment, you might remember that he was really worried that he'd harm people. Let's put that worry into the revolving door ...

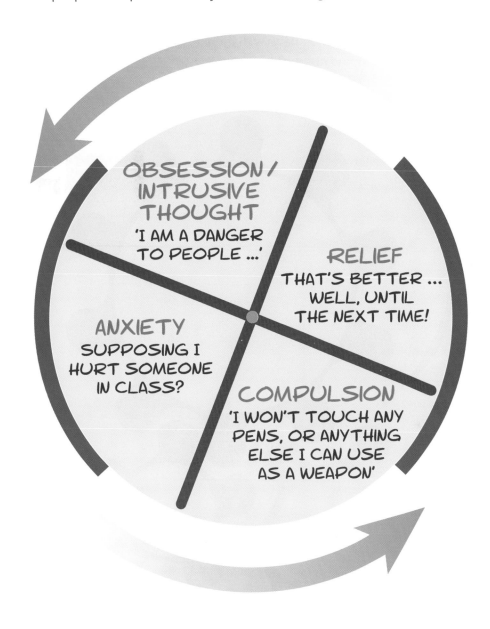

Okay, now it's your turn to take your worry on a trip in the revolving door! Have a look at the diagram below and fill in the gaps to help you understand what's going on for you …

So now you can see how this 'revolving door' of obsessions and compulsions is stopping you from finding the exit sign. But the good news is that the exit sign really is there – and in the next chapter we'll show you how to find it!

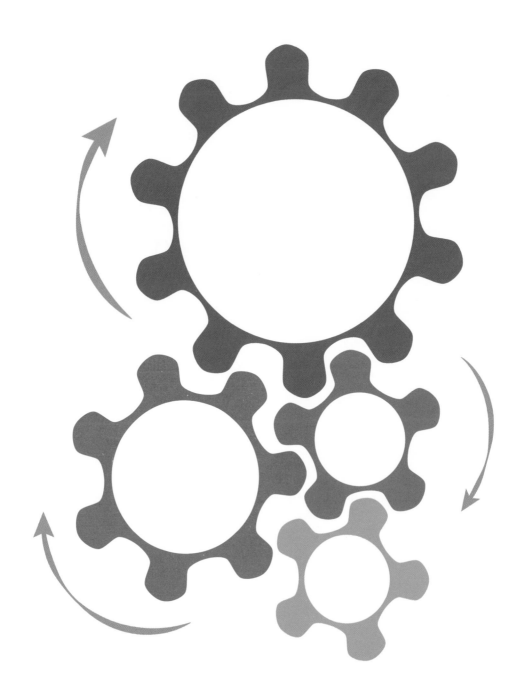

Chapter 23

Recovery from OCD

Just take a breather for a second. You've already come a really long way. So I think you should give yourself some serious respect for getting this far. By reading this book you've taken huge steps to manage your OCD and anxiety and you should congratulate yourself for that.

Now, we're going to give you the tools you need to recover from OCD. In the last chapter we looked at the 'One Hand' and the 'Other Hand' test to help you find out which is the true version of the story. Next we're going to tell you more about the **'Accept-Embrace-Control'** technique. If you've already read the 'Teenagers' section, you'll already know these techniques; they work equally well for OCD. In this chapter, we'll also look at some other techniques that work well for obsessions and compulsions. I don't think you'll find any of them too difficult for you, and I know they can really help you.

These techniques are:

- The Two Hands Theory. This helps you look at your worry from different points of view.
- Climbing the Worry Ladder. Take it one step at a time, and see how far you get.
- Changing Scenarios. Where you can or can't change the future.
- Shifting Your Attention by first focusing on your worry, then looking at a familiar object and describing it in detail.
- The responsibility pie chart. This helps you see who might really be responsible for the things you're worrying about.
- Helpful Distractions. Find a way to relax, and help you recover.

DON'T HIDE IT - TALK ABOUT IT

This is one of the best things you can do to kick-start your recovery. Now, I know that this sounds difficult, but please, **REMEMBER** ...

A problem shared is a problem halved. Even though you're reading this book, you still might be finding it very difficult to tell anyone about your OCD. Perhaps you feel guilty about the kind of thoughts, or sensations, or images you're experiencing. Perhaps you're ashamed and embarrassed to admit you're having difficulties. You might also be worried about what people will think of you if you tell them ...

Please don't worry! **There is nothing to be ashamed of.**

Everybody experiences anxiety at some stage in their lives, and everyone has intrusive thoughts. **Both these things are completely normal.**

Adam told me that he had intrusive thoughts about harming people. He wasn't a violent person – and he certainly didn't want to hurt anyone. So these thoughts made him feel very guilty and scared. Unfortunately, he couldn't let the thoughts go, and he didn't feel that he could tell anyone about them. So the intrusive thoughts kept coming back, making his life miserable.

A friend of mine told me about a trip she'd taken in a hot air balloon. It was actually her third balloon flight, so she was quite used to the experience, but she told me she'd suddenly thought, 'What if I sit on the edge of the basket and push myself off?' My friend was happy in her life, and had no wish to commit suicide. It was simply a random thought, and fortunately, she was able to let it go.

Adam couldn't let go of his thoughts so easily. And perhaps you feel the same. But please believe me when I say, just because your worries have turned into a problem, it doesn't mean to say they will be around for ever. By telling a parent, a family member, a teacher or someone else you trust, you will be taking another big step towards tackling your difficulties

Think back to Adam's story…

'I didn't tell my parents as I thought they wouldn't understand, and I daren't go to the doctor in case I was diagnosed as 'mad' and sent to a mental hospital. For me, it seemed the only option was to sort it out myself.'

Did keeping the problem to himself help Adam? Did he manage to sort it out alone? The answer to both questions is 'No'. And because he didn't tell anyone, or couldn't make someone understand him, his problems lasted well into his adulthood.

Unluckily for Adam, his OCD was around at a time when disorders like his weren't understood as well as they are now. Today, there is a lot more understanding of OCD and the nature of the illness, as well as good treatment for people like you.

So if you're suffering, PLEASE TELL SOMEONE!

You can take a copy of this book to show them. Even if the person you tell doesn't quite 'get it', they will probably be able to point you in the direction of someone who can. Please remember that there are so many people who can help you and want to help you.

ACCEPT-EMBRACE-CONTROL

Okay, so let's have a look at some techniques to help you get a handle on your OCD. If you've read Chapters 17–21, you'll recall that our recovery approach falls into three areas: 'Accept', 'Embrace' and 'Control'. Here are three statements which help to explain each one:

- **ACCEPT** that you – like the rest of us – sometimes have weird / unusual / upsetting and uncontrollable intrusions (thoughts, doubts, images, sensations, urges), and that is a completely normal situation. It's not the thought that counts – it's the importance and the meaning we attach to the thought. For example, thinking we are 100 per cent responsible (a 'me to the rescue' thinking trap) for making sure something does / doesn't happen. Or thinking the **worst-case scenario** will definitely happen. We must remember, thoughts are only thoughts …

- **EMBRACE** those thoughts, worries and anxieties. By this, we mean face up to them and challenge them using the one hand / other hand technique, so you can see them for what they are.

- **CONTROL** your OCD by continuing your experiments, not judging your intrusions and being kind to yourself.

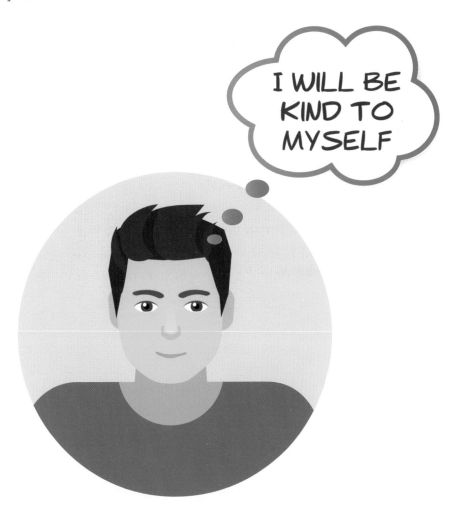

ARE YOU REALLY THAT RESPONSIBLE?

If your OCD is making you think you are 100 per cent responsible for preventing something awful from happening, for example an accident or spreading a terrible illness, first apply the Two Hands test to work out whether the OCD worry is realistic (or whether it is just a worry problem!) and whether you are actually the only person responsible for stopping something awful from happening. Here's an example for you to look at before you work on your own OCD worry.

ON THE 'ONE HAND' ...

my problem is that I will cause my ill grandmother to die by passing on some germs from not washing my hands.

WHAT WAYS AM I MAKING SURE THAT THIS DOESN'T COME TRUE, AND WHAT ELSE DO I NEED TO BE DOING TO MAKE SURE IT DOESN'T COME TRUE:

- Washing my hands all the time! (Like the signs at the hospital)
- Avoid going to places that might be dirty or unhygienic
- Not visit my grandmother in hospital just in case
- Making sure that my family also wash their hands all the time
- Taking longer showers so I can wash myself properly
- Change my clothes when I come in from school or being outside so I don't spread germs at home

EVIDENCE FOR THIS POSITION BEING TRUE:

- Germs cause illness
- The signs at the hospital say to wash your hands before going in to the wards so it must be important
- Old people are more likely to get sick

ON THE 'OTHER HAND' ...

My problem is that I worry I'll spread germs, but there is not way of knowing as I can't actually see the germs, and I just want my grandmother to be okay.

IF THIS POSITION IS TRUE, WHAT DO I NEED TO BE DOING:

- I need to stop worrying and can wash my hands as much as other people
- Visit my grandmother in hospital

EVIDENCE FOR THIS POSITION BEING TRUE:

- I can't see germs so there is no way of knowing whether I have any on me
- I worry about lots of other things too so it is likely to be a worry problem
- I've only just started washing my hands a lot but previously I didn't think about germs so much and no one (including me) got ill and died ... so it can't be about germs
- My family visit my grandmother and no one else thinks about germs as much as me, but they wouldn't want to cause my grandmother to get more ill
- If spreading germs was such a big problem they wouldn't let anyone visit hospitals
- Other people don't think about this as much as me, but don't want to spread germs unnecessarily to their families either, so it must be me worrying about it

BASED ON THE EVIDENCE, WHICH POSITION DO YOU THINK IS MORE LIKELY TO BE TRUE?

ON THE 'ONE HAND' MY PROBLEM IS ...

_____

_____

_____

WHAT WAYS AM I MAKING SURE THAT THIS DOESN'T COME TRUE, AND WHAT
ELSE DO I NEED TO BE DOING TO MAKE SURE IT DOESN'T COME TRUE:

_____

_____

_____

EVIDENCE FOR THIS POSITION BEING TRUE:

_____

_____

_____

_____

_____

_____

_____

ON THE 'OTHER HAND' MY PROBLEM IS THAT I WORRY THAT ...

_____

_____

_____

_____

WHAT WAYS AM I MAKING SURE THAT THIS DOESN'T COME TRUE, AND WHAT
ELSE DO I NEED TO BE DOING TO MAKE SURE IT DOESN'T COME TRUE:

_____

_____

_____

EVIDENCE FOR THIS POSITION BEING TRUE:

_____

_____

_____

_____

_____

_____

BASED ON THE EVIDENCE, WHICH POSITION DO YOU THINK IS MORE LIKELY
TO BE TRUE?

Then, if you think that other people you think might share responsibility note them down here and how much responsibility they have. If you can't think of anyone else who you believe might be responsible to stop these things from happening, then is most likely to be that no-one is responsible and down to change or bad luck, as sometimes in life unfortunate things happen.

Next, fill in the pie chart below, dividing it between all those who might also be 'responsible' for the thing you're worrying about ...

Okay, you've now taken a very big step towards **accepting** that the thoughts, images, doubts, sensations and urges which are still upsetting / intrusive / weird / controlling – are just thoughts. Your OCD is making them seem bigger / more important / scarier than they already are.

Your OCD is telling you something that isn't really true!

Okay, hopefully that's helped you to accept what is really going on for you.

This is a problem of worrying about your thought / feeling / image / urge, not what your OCD is telling you it is.

Over the next few pages we've set some experiments that will help you to **embrace** your OCD and anxiety. While you're doing the experiments, it's worthwhile keeping a diary of your life with OCD, what it makes you do, and for how long.

Remember Abbie? She thought she was 100 per cent responsible for looking after the safety of the school's computer room. Here is an extract from her diary.

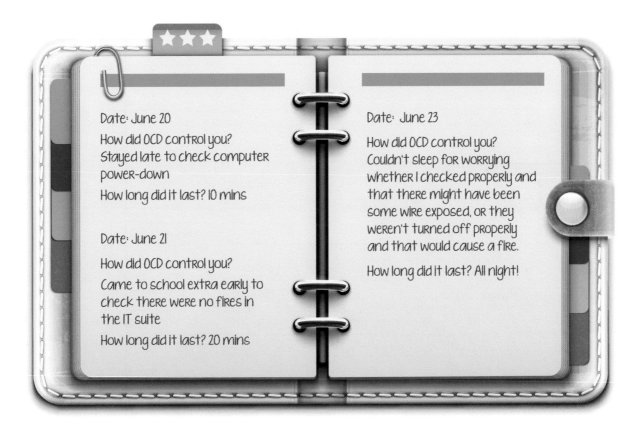

Keeping a diary like this is a very useful way of seeing your obsessions and compulsions in black and white. It might also be useful for the future, when you look back and think, 'Wow – was that really happening to me? I'm so glad it isn't happening now!'

Then, make a list of all the other people you think might share responsibility and how much responsibility they have. For example, in the case of Annie above who worried about spreading germs and causing her grandmother in hospital to die, she might include all the people responsible for keeping her grandmother well such as doctors and nurses, and other family members.

JUGGLING BALLS

'Okay,' you might say, 'I have a lot of compulsions. And they all feel scary! Which one should I tackle first?'

Good question. We've heard about Abbie, and you've read some of her diary extracts. When I asked Abbie how she would feel if she didn't check and re-check them, she said it would be too difficult at first not to stay after school to check that the computers had been powered down. However, she did agree that because the caretaker came in to school at 7.30am, she might be able to manage not getting into school early to check about possible fires in the IT suite.

We came to this agreement by using the idea of **rubber balls** and **glass balls**. This is a military technique for prioritising tasks, but it's very useful for tackling compulsions too:

- 'Rubber balls' were OCD worries that could be dropped safely.
- 'Glass balls' were still OCD worries but ones that still felt precious, and couldn't be dropped without worrying about the consequences.

This is part of Abbie's 'rubber balls / glass balls' chart …

OCD PROBLEMS	RUBBER BALL OR GLASS BALL?
1) Checking computers at night	A) Glass
2) Checking computers in the morning	A) Rubber
3) Monitoring students for IT misuse	A) Glass
4) Praying to God that nothing will happen	A) Rubber
5) Constantly cleaning dust off keyboards	A) Bit of both!

By weighing up her OCD problems using the 'rubber balls / glass balls' technique, Abbie was starting to see some of her difficulties more objectively; that is, she was seeing her thoughts for what they were – just thoughts. And she didn't feel pressured into dropping her 'glass balls' before she felt ready to turn them into rubber ones!

Maybe you could try this exercise? On the following page, fill in your compulsions and rate them 'rubber ball' or 'glass ball'. Then have a think about which of the rubber balls you feel you could 'drop' first – i.e. which you would like to tackle using the experiments in the next few days. Remember that some rubber balls disguise themselves as glass balls (to avoid being dropped), and eventually we will have to drop these too if they don't change into obvious rubber balls.

Before you carry out your experiment, check in with how you feel now ...

BEFORE THE EXPERIMENT, I FEEL ...

I worry that... _____

_____

_____

I feel... _____

_____

MY OCD PROBLEMS ARE   RUBBER BALL OR GLASS BALL?

- _____
- _____
- _____
- _____
- _____

Repeating these experiments, and going a little further each time, is by far the best way of tackling your OCD. If you feel uncomfortable, please keep going – because that means you're doing it right! Remember that we're embracing OCD, not forcing it to slink off into a corner so that it can come back even stronger. It's a bit like making friends with someone you used to think was a bully – when you discover what lies beneath that person, you wonder why you were ever afraid of him or her. When OCD shows how vulnerable it is, that is the time to take back any power it had over you.

Let's have a look at Abbie's experiment ...

ABBIE'S EXPERIMENT

MY EXPERIMENT IS TO ...
see if I can stop going into school early to check for fires in the IT department.

ON THE ONE HAND ...
OCD tells me if I don't go in, there will be a fire.

ON THE OTHER HAND ...
I'm worrying there will be a fire but it is unlikely and even if it happened, it wouldn't be my fault. This is a worry problem!

MY EXPERIMENT, AND THE TWO HANDS TEST

MY EXPERIMENT IS TO ...

_____

_____

ON THE ONE HAND ...

_____

_____

_____

ON THE OTHER HAND ...

_____

_____

_____

_____

So that was Abbie's experiment challenge. In the box above, write down yours, and fill in your thoughts about the 'One Hand' and the 'Other Hand' theories.

How did you get on? Did it make you feel less anxious about doing your own experiment? If so, give it a go now. Remember – set big goals, but take small steps towards them, and don't worry if you feel uncomfortable about doing them. That is natural – and it means you're really pushing yourself. But each time you do the experiment, you will feel less anxious. And remember ... this is a problem of worrying about your thought / sensations / doubts / image / urges, as opposed to what your OCD is telling you it is!

Okay, so hopefully now you've given your experiment a go. How did you get on? If you felt uncomfortable, then that shows you were doing it correctly. Did it turn out the way your worries told you it might, or did something else happen?

Let's look at Abbie's feedback ...

Q: DID THE 'ONE HAND' PREDICTION COME TRUE?

A: No. There was no fire!!!

Q: HOW DID YOU FEEL?

A: Very anxious when 7.30am came around, but I just tried to get on with getting ready for school which helped.

Q: IF THE 'OTHER HAND' POSITION IS THAT YOU HAVE A WORRY-BASED PROBLEM THAT MAKES YOU ANXIOUS IS TRUE, WHAT SHOULD YOU DO NOW?

A: Stop worrying! Take my time to go to school and leave on time.

Q: WHAT DID YOU LEARN FROM THIS EXPERIMENT?

A: That it is a worry problem and I need to work on my worry. It's not a problem of fires or other issues with the equipment.

Q: IS YOUR WORRY STILL THERE?

A: Yes, because I still feel somewhat responsible for the safety of the IT department.

Q: HOW CAN YOU EXPERIMENT WITH THIS?

A: To see what happens when I don't stay behind to turn off all the machines.

Now, fill in the box below with you own experience:

Q: WHAT HAPPENED?

Q: HOW DID YOU FEEL?

Q: DID THE 'ONE HAND' PREDICTION COME TRUE?

Q: IF THE 'OTHER HAND' POSITION IS THAT YOU HAVE A WORRY-BASED PROBLEM THAT MAKES YOU ANXIOUS IS TRUE, WHAT SHOULD YOU DO NOW?

Q: WHAT DID YOU LEARN FROM THIS EXPERIMENT?

Q: IS YOUR WORRY STILL THERE?

Q: HOW CAN YOU EXPERIMENT WITH THIS?

OCD - YOU'RE NOT THE BOSS OF ME!

We encourage you to embrace OCD by doing the experiments and seeing your worries for what they are. Sometimes it's good to remind OCD that it's no longer in charge, and let it know that it can't push you around.

While Abbie was doing her experiments, she felt it was important to tell her OCD exactly what she thought of it. When she did this, it made her feel more powerful and in charge. I asked her to write down what she'd like to say to her OCD. Here's what she said:

1) *OCD back off! You're not going to worry me any more!*

2) *You think you're strong, but we all know, you're the loser here.*

3) *I know you're trying to trick me, but you didn't manage it today, did you? Nice try!!*

4) *Talk to the hand, OCD!*

5) *Think you're clever? Sorry – I'm way smarter than you!*

If you could give your OCD a talking-to, what would you say?! Below, write five strong statements directly to your OCD:

1)

2)

3)

4)

5)

When we're doing this, it's important to know that we're NOT turning it into another ritual, another way of hiding from OCD. We're not doing this to reduce our anxiety. We are doing this to make ourselves feel more positive. We are doing this to put OCD firmly in its place.

Up to this point, we've given you a lot of tools that will help you to Accept and Embrace OCD. Now we're going to talk about Controlling it. As we mentioned, the way to control your OCD is by learning NOT to control it.

Confused?!

CONTROL, NOT FIGHT

It might sound strange, but this is exactly the right approach. Instead of fighting OCD and anxiety, we take control of it by allowing it in. Every time you accept and embrace, you reduce the power OCD has over you and keep on reducing it until it becomes a tiny little voice in the background that you can easily ignore.

'What's the evidence for this?' you might ask. 'Why should I accept OCD, after all this time I've spent fighting it?'

Fair question. But ask yourself this. Did all that 'fight' achieve anything? Did it lessen your OCD, or make it go away altogether? Sadly, the answer is 'NO', because OCD is smart, and knows all the tricks people use to fight it.

But the one thing it really doesn't like is when you accept and embrace it for what it is – just a collection of unwanted, intrusive thoughts that don't mean anything. And if you look at OCD this way, you are far, far smarter than it will ever be!

It's perfectly normal if the progress of your recovery goes up and down – but being kind to yourself will really help you to go beyond your difficulties with OCD. Please try some of the relaxation techniques we gave you in this chapter, and make sure you make time for all the things you enjoy in life. Keep on having fun and getting out – keep on doing the things you want to do even if you sometimes feel like you don't want to.

As we've said, there will be times during your recovery that OCD will try to take control again. That's not surprising; it has been a powerful force in your life, and it would like to be the boss again. You might also find that it jumps from one thing you've obsessed about (and managed to sort out) onto something unexpected; something you didn't see coming.

SMART THINKING

Again, the way to deal with this is to be smarter than OCD. Have a think back, and remind yourself of:

- What intrusions and obsessions are. We know that they're uncontrollable and unwanted thoughts, images, urges, doubts and sensations.
- What 'compulsions' are ...
- ... And how the two work together to create the disorder.
- What the 'Thinking Traps' are, including 'Me to the Rescue' (where you assume 100 per cent responsibility for everything) and Worst-Case Scenario (where you assume the worst ending will always happen) and how you fall into them.
- The One Hand / Other Hand theory and how to examine the evidence for your intrusions.
- Other experiments you can do, for example, the Worry Ladder.
- Helpful distractions.
- Relaxation.

Understanding how OCD works and what you can do about it is the key to dealing with any new problems that might arise. Don't try to avoid your OCD, or do anything to make it go away quickly – because we all know what happens when you do that! Instead, walk towards the problem, carry out some new experiments, be brave and be bold, accept and embrace OCD, and take control once again.

If we look back to Adam's story, we can see that his recovery took time, and there were ups and downs along the way. He knows how helpful it is to tell someone about your OCD and anxieties. So please – if you're struggling to maintain your recovery and you feel OCD is taking over your life again, make sure you tell someone. A parent, a teacher, a learning mentor, or just someone you trust. All these people can help you, and even if they don't quite know what's going on for you, they can recommend that you see your local doctor, a qualified CBT therapist, or a psychologist like me. You don't have to suffer alone any more – help is always out there!

CHAPTER SUMMARY

- OCD is an **obsessional problem that can be about anything, causing us to feel anxious, depressed, disgusted, ashamed and guilty**. In brief, OCD is when people have intrusions that are very upsetting, which they interpret to be very threatening, so they feel worried, anxious and fearful, and naturally want to minimise or reduce the threat.

- With OCD, you interpret the intrusive thought as being 'doom and gloom', and so you feel compelled to carry out rituals because you feel responsible for preventing the bad thing from happening (that's a 'me to the rescue' thinking trap).

- With OCD it's NOT the thought that counts – it's the importance and meaning we give to it, and the compulsions (rituals, avoidance, safety behaviours, etc.) we do to make ourselves feel better.

- By using the One Hand and Other Hand method, the responsibility pie chart and the other techniques and experiments we've shown you, you can try telling yourself a different story about your thoughts, doubts, images, sensations and urges.

- When you Accept and Embrace the worries and anxieties which cause your OCD (by letting them in and not running from them), you will come to learn how OCD works. The more you experiment, the less anxious you will feel.

Chapter 24

Panic Attacks

You might have found that, as part of your emotional and bodily reaction to your anxiety or OCD, you have experienced a **panic attack**. This is a feeling of terror that strikes suddenly, sometimes without warning, and sometimes in a situation that you know is going to be scary. It's like that moment in a horror movie when you wished you'd shut your eyes. You feel out of control, and worry that something terrible might happen to you. You might experience:

- Palpitations (heart beating quickly)
- Sweating
- Trembling and shaking
- Shortness of breath
- Feelings of choking
- Chest pain
- Feeling sick
- Dizziness
- Numbness
- Fear of dying
- Feelings that you will lose control of your bowels or bladder

WHAT PANIC LOOKS LIKE

Here is a model of panic attacks, which we have reproduced with the permission of the author, Professor David Clark[4]:

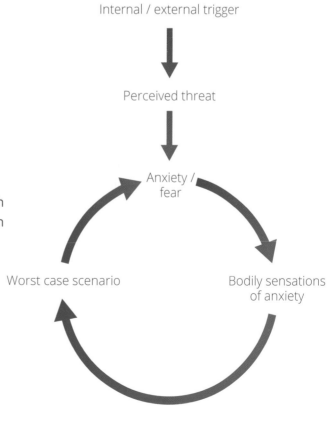

Model of panic

Internal / external trigger

Perceived threat

Anxiety / fear

Bodily sensations of anxiety

Worst case scenario

Figure 8: Cognitive model of panic.

A panic attack is started by a trigger. That trigger could be suddenly confronting your worst fear without warning, or a thought that pops into your head which suddenly spins out of control. You'll probably feel a physical sensation – perhaps your hands will tingle or your heart rate will jump – and your Worst-Case Scenario **interpretation of events** is that something very dangerous is happening to your body. Some common thoughts, related to the sensations you're feeling include, 'Am I going mad?' 'Will I wet myself?' 'Am I going to pass out?' 'Will I do something embarrassing?' These interpretations (or misinterpretations) make you anxious. In turn, this increases the severity of the symptoms you're feeling. It's a very hard cycle to break. But we can help you.

First of all, you need to know that, even though it feels absolutely awful, what is happening in your body is actually completely normal. In a panic attack, your body goes into 'fight, flight or freeze' mode as a response to something that is making you anxious. So all those feelings you might experience when you're having a panic attack – the increased heart rate, shortness of breath, feeling hot and sweaty, blurry vision, sensations of choking, and tingling feelings – they're all completely normal.

Will remembering that make you feel better the next time you have a panic attack?! Probably not!

'Okay,' you might argue, 'it's easy to say panic attacks are completely normal when you're not having one. When you ARE having one it feels like the most frightening thing on earth!' I know it does. And that's why people who have panic attacks go to such great lengths to avoid them. You might carry around 'rescue remedies', paper bags (to breathe into), bottles of water, tablets and toilet paper in the hope that these will help in the event of an attack. These are what we'd describe as 'safety behaviours', and we have already seen how people use them to avoid worry, anxiety and OCD. But just like worry, anxiety and OCD, by avoiding panic attacks, you make the fear of them even worse, and that spins the 'Worry Wheel' faster and faster.

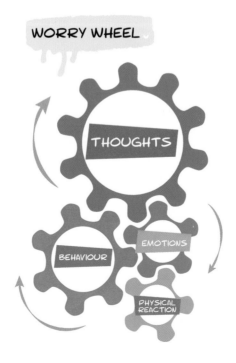

WORRY WHEEL

THOUGHTS

BEHAVIOUR

EMOTIONS

PHYSICAL REACTION

There are a number of physical sensations you may experience associated with the physiological changes in the body due to the fight, flight or freeze response.

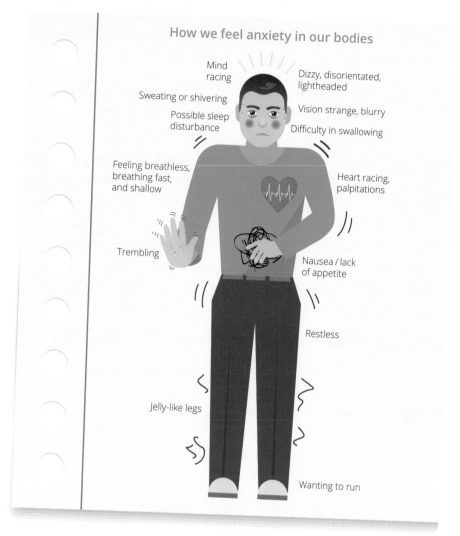

How we feel anxiety in our bodies

Mind racing

Dizzy, disorientated, lightheaded

Sweating or shivering

Vision strange, blurry

Possible sleep disturbance

Difficulty in swallowing

Feeling breathless, breathing fast, and shallow

Heart racing, palpitations

Trembling

Nausea / lack of appetite

Restless

Jelly-like legs

Wanting to run

SO WHAT CAN YOU DO ABOUT IT?

Let's ask Zara about the time she had a panic attack:

'I'm Zara, I'm 14, and I get anxious if I feel that I'll get trapped somewhere. A few months ago I agreed to go to the cinema with my friend. Halfway through the movie I felt a really weird feeling coming on. It was like I couldn't breathe; I felt really sick and shaky and I don't know how I managed to get out of the cinema without fainting. So I went to the doctor, told her what had happened and she said it was a panic attack. Ever since then I've tried to avoid places that are closed in, so I don't go to the mall with my friends any more, and I even have difficulties sitting in the classroom. I carry rescue remedies and paper bags with me at all times. I'm really scared of it happening again.'

Now she knows she had a panic attack, Zara is scared of having another one. We can see why she is scared of having another one. Even though we know it's a bodily reaction, and that it will pass, it doesn't mean to say that it doesn't feel real.

HOW TO EMBRACE PANIC

Hiding from panic attacks isn't the way to make sure they don't happen. By now, you might be able to guess the solution ... that's right ... you need to accept and embrace them!

'How can I possibly embrace a panic attack?' you might ask. 'They're horrible and weird and scary! They're worse than anything!'

Yes, they are scary. But ask yourself these questions:

When I last had a panic attack did I:

- Go mad?
- Faint
- Do something embarrassing?
- Lose control of my bowels / bladder?
- End up in hospital?
- Experience my own worst-case scenario?

I'm betting that none of these things happened, and that the panic attack eventually passed. So what you believed might happen didn't happen. In that case, we can consider another interpretation about panic attacks, one which is based more on reality than the **'Worst-Case Thinking Trap'** that you are imagining ...

CHANGING THE WAY WE THINK ABOUT PANIC ATTACKS

We know from Adam's story that he suffered lots of panic attacks. Things got so bad that he actually thought he was going mad. And that's not really surprising; people who have regular panic attacks can't just carry on their life as normal after an attack has passed; they live in fear of the next one striking. And the one after that and so on ... It is exhausting.

But we can challenge this belief. If you suffer from panic attacks, you're not going mad, I promise. Try asking yourself these questions:

> *Q: How many times have you had a panic attack in the past year?*
> *A: Approximately ten times per month.*
>
> *Q: So that's approximately 120 panic attacks this year?*
> *A: Yes, that's right.*
>
> *Q: Have you gone mad?*
> *A: No.*
>
> *Q: Have you had to go to a psychiatric hospital?*
> *A: No.*
>
> *Q: Has life gone back to normal following the attack?*
> *A: Yes.*
>
> *Q: How many people do you know have gone mad through panic attacks?*
> *A: None.*

Based on these answers, what do you think are the chances that you will go mad as a result of a panic attack?

ON THE OTHER HAND ...

Let's try the One Hand / Other Hand test to look at another common worry. Meet Ben. Ben is 15. When he was in an exam a few months ago, Ben felt really stressed. He knew he could do well in the exam, but it didn't feel like it was going as well as he'd hoped. He started to feel more and more uncomfortable sitting in the same place for so long, and felt that he was shaking very badly. He didn't know what to do, and he was too scared to put his hand up to be excused because his body felt 'wrong'. He had a feeling that he would pass out or do something else really embarrassing, and he felt like he needed to go to the toilet before he wet himself. Ben felt incredibly self-conscious, hot and uncomfortable, and he felt as if everyone could tell that he was desperate for the toilet.

Since the exam, Ben has had the same feelings in other situations. When he went to football with his dad, he was stuck in the middle of a row of people. When he started to experience the strange feelings again, he knew it would be difficult to find his way out to the toilet if he needed to go. By the middle of the second half, he was convinced that he was going to lose control of his bladder and wet himself. But he didn't feel like he could get up and make his way out, so he carried on sitting there, feeling more and more stressed about the situation. After the match Ben ran to the toilet, but found that he didn't actually need to pee very badly after all.

Ben has since found out about panic attacks. And he has experienced them in several other situations.

Let's review his thoughts ...

ON THE 'ONE HAND' ...
I get really stressed thinking that I will lose control of my body, and wet myself when I have a panic attack ...

ON THE 'OTHER HAND' ...
My body is going through a natural 'fight, flight or freeze' process and while I find it very uncomfortable, it is in fact a normal experience and not dangerous, and will pass soon.

EVIDENCE FOR THIS POSITION BEING TRUE ...
- When I'm in a stressful situation, I start to feel like I'm going to lose control of my body and my bladder. The feeling gets so bad that I start to panic more and more.

EVIDENCE FOR THIS POSITION BEING TRUE ...
- I have had lots of panic attacks over the past six months and while they're horrible, I've never wet myself or done anything embarrassing.
  In addition, panic attacks are an anxiety response, and anxiety is a normal human experience.

WHAT ABOUT YOU?

If you've had a panic attack I'm guessing that it passed without any physical danger to you, or any embarrassing consequences, and while it felt very uncomfortable and frightening, it was no more serious than that. So changing your own story (your interpretation) of how you see the panic attack is really important – only then will you be able to accept and embrace what is happening, and let those feelings be while not avoiding them.

When I was a student, I once spent a whole night working on a project that had to be handed in the following day. I didn't sleep, and drank a lot of coffee. On the way into college the next day, I had a panic attack. It was very unpleasant and scary and I might have also thought that I was going mad, or might have a heart attack.

But I knew it was nothing to do with any of that.

Instead, I chose to see it as my body's way of dealing with the fact that I hadn't slept, and had had too much caffeine. I was wired and I was feeling anxious about getting the paper in on time. I knew my experience was unpleasant, but I also knew it wasn't 'Worst-Case Scenario'. The panic attack soon passed.

Let's have a look at how worry over panic attacks is affecting your life. Ask yourself these questions and write your answers in the boxes below:

WHAT ARE THE THINGS I HAVE STOPPED DOING IN CASE I HAVE A PANIC ATTACK?
(For example, stopping going to the movies, using public transport etc.)

WHAT PLACES HAVE I STOPPED VISITING IN CASE I HAVE A PANIC ATTACK?
(For example, places that might be crowded or those you can't 'escape' from quickly)

WHAT THINGS HAVE I STARTED DOING TO MAKE SURE I DON'T HAVE A PANIC ATTACK? (For example, making sure you always have water, a bag to breathe into, or you know where the bathrooms are in public places)

So now you can see how your **worry** about panic attacks is affecting your life, what can you do to accept, embrace and ultimately control it? Just as with worry, anxiety, and OCD, you need to test out your reaction to panic attacks by experimenting with it. Below is the experiment we set for Zara:

MY 'WORST-CASE THINKING TRAP' INTERPRETATION IS THAT IF I HAVE A PANIC ATTACK, I WILL FAINT AND BE TAKEN TO HOSPITAL.

WHAT DOES THE EVIDENCE SAY?

Panic attacks are extreme episodes of anxiety but they are not dangerous and I don't need to go to hospital.

MY EXPERIMENT IS:

To allow myself to have a panic attack if I feel it start to happen. I will go somewhere I have avoided because I'm scared that it might cause a panic attack. So I will go to the mall on my own for 10 minutes, without my paper bag or rescue remedies and see what happens.

WHAT SAFETY BEHAVIOURS WILL I NOT DO?

I won't take my paper bag or any other rescue remedies with me and stop avoiding places and situations that I worry about.

WHAT HAPPENED?

I was very nervous and I felt a panic attack coming on. So I waited until it had passed. It wasn't nice, but I didn't have to go to hospital!

WHAT SHOULD I DO NEXT?

I could go to the mall for longer next time. I could eventually plan another cinema visit with my friends.

Although it wasn't nice for Zara to experience the feelings of a panic attack, she did the right thing by accepting and embracing it. By doing this, she regained some of the power that the fear of panic attacks had over her, and now she feels confident to face her fear again.

In the box on the next page, write down where your fear of panic attacks lies, and what you can do about it …

MY 'WORST-CASE THINKING TRAP' INTERPRETATION IS THAT IF I HAVE A PANIC ATTACK, I WILL ...

WHAT DOES THE EVIDENCE SAY?

_____

_____

_____

MY EXPERIMENT IS:

_____

_____

_____

WHAT SAFETY BEHAVIOURS WILL I NOT DO?

_____

_____

_____

_____

_____

WHAT HAPPENED?

_____

_____

_____

WHAT SHOULD I DO NEXT?

_____

_____

YOUR NEXT STEPS TOWARDS BEATING PANIC

Okay, hopefully you can now see what the 'threat' from panic attacks really is (just your body's response) and how this fear is driving the Worry Wheel. You now know how to slow down or stop that wheel by accepting and embracing panic attacks.

We have looked at ways you can review the thoughts that accompany a panic attack and challenge your Worst-Case Scenario thinking. You have strategies that you can use straightaway … but I know that the thought of having another panic attack may still be scary! So if it is, do your experiments in stages, just like Zara did. Do you remember the Worry Ladder we talked about?

If not, take a look back and see how you can accept and embrace panic attacks by taking one step at a time up the Worry Ladder. Visit the place or situation you feel might give you a panic attack – but for no more than 10 minutes at first. Don't take any of the 'equipment' (the rescue remedies, pills, water or paper bags) that you might otherwise use as a 'safety behaviour' in the event of a panic attack. Gradually build it up until you can stay there for half an hour without feeling any of the symptoms of a panic attack.

By embracing panic attacks in this way, you will discover that you regain control over your life. Panic attacks won't be able to control you – or put any more restrictions on how you live your life.

Chapter 25

A Plan for Life Beyond OCD, Anxiety, and Worry

Now we've worked through Anxiety, Worry, and OCD, let's look at how we can maintain good mental health in the future.

We've spent a long time looking at ways you can confront your expectations and embrace your OCD. But now we're going to take a different perspective ...

It's surprising how big an impact food and diet can have on your mental health. As his depression took hold, Adam went from being fit and sporty to being overweight. Fighting against OCD and anxiety can be so tiring that it leaves no room for anything else. Without the energy to get out of bed, Adam stopped looking after himself, stopped exercising and started drinking too many sugary fizzy drinks and relying on junk food.

Maybe you've tried to keep yourself going with energy drinks or comfort food? The problem with these things is that they can only improve your mood very briefly. When the effects wear off, you're likely to feel even worse than you did before.

If you've ever seen a doctor about your battles with anxiety, depression, and OCD, they probably told you to get some exercise. You might even be sick of hearing people tell you to get out and get some fresh air. But, I have to tell you ... exercise really does work.

Okay, it won't 'cure' your feelings, but even a bit of gentle exercise, especially outdoors, helps produce and release serotonin in your system. And serotonin helps regulate our mood. Just 10–15 minutes' exercise every day – brisk walking is fine – can help change the way you feel.

It might not feel easy at first. If you have anxiety around getting out and being seen in public, you might have to work through your One Hand / Other Hand technique.

- Pick an activity you'll enjoy – any activity is good – walking, running, swimming, football, climbing ...
- Start small. Just getting out is a good start. You can step up the time you exercise day by day, or even week by week if you prefer.
- Give it time. You won't feel better straightaway, but if you keep at it, you WILL notice the positive effects. The exercise will make you feel more relaxed and calm.
- Keep pushing. When five minutes feels comfortable, try ten. When 1 kilometre feels easy, try 2 kilometres.
- Remember that effective exercise depends on good nutrition ...

YOU ARE WHAT YOU EAT

Eating a healthy balanced diet doesn't have to be hard work. And you don't have to cut out your favourite treats altogether. My advice is, be sensible, but be kind to yourself too!

HERE ARE SOME POINTERS:

You probably already know that you're supposed to have a minimum of five fruit and veg a day. It sounds like a lot – but it's not so bad. Baked beans on toast is one portion, a piece of fruit is another, a few tablespoons of peas or sweetcorn is a portion. Vegetables that go into other foods count too – e.g. the onion that you use for seasoning and the tinned tomatoes in a spaghetti bolognese.

- Rewards are good. If you eat well in the week, it's good to have a treat at the weekend – and I bet, it'll taste all the better for waiting.
- Try and cut down on fizzy drinks and energy drinks – they're full of caffeine and sugar.
- Learn how to cook. Some people find that cooking for themselves helps them to eat better. It can be relaxing too.
- You need a good mix of foods to keep your body and mind functioning well, e.g.:
  - Starchy food like rice, pasta and potatoes to make you feel fuller for longer.
  - Protein helps our brain function, builds muscle and makes antibodies to keep you well (it also makes us feel full for longer). Eggs, milk, fish, pistachio nuts, chicken, turkey, beans and pulses are all good sources of protein.
  - Drink plenty of fluids, especially water – it's got zero calories and will refresh you better than anything else.

YOUR STAYING WELL PLAN

So, we've looked at many ways in which you can challenge your anxieties and OCD, so if you feel them creeping up again, take a deep breath and work through all the strategies we've shown you. You can also try this Prevention and Maintenance chart. If you feel your OCD or anxiety starting to return, just fill it in ...

WHAT IS YOUR ANXIETY / OCD DOING TO BOTHER YOU?

WHAT DID YOU DO TO TRY AND BEAT IT?

HOW DID THAT GO?

NOW YOU UNDERSTAND IT, WHAT WORKED FOR YOU TO HELP GET ON TOP OF IT?

IF YOUR ANXIETY / OCD RETURNS WHAT CAN YOU DO TO TRY TO CHALLENGE IT?

This next bit is really important – please don't forget to be kind to yourself!

Right back at the beginning, we asked you to write down some positive things about yourself and what people like about you. Now, after all you've done and all that you're starting to achieve, use the space below to write down what you're most proud of about what you've achieved in working through this book.

I WAS MOST PROUD OF ...

_____

_____

_____

_____

Okay, now you've done that, let's create a plan that will keep you well, and help you if you ever feel your anxiety or OCD coming back. If it helps, make a copy of this page, so you've got it close to hand whenever you need it.

THE SIGNS THAT MY ANXIETY / OCD IS COMING BACK ARE:

_____

_____

_____

_____

_____

WHEN THIS HAPPENS, MY NEXT MOVE WILL BE TO:

_____

_____

_____

_____

_____

_____

_____

I WILL PROTECT MYSELF BY:

_____

_____

_____

_____

_____

IT WILL ALSO BE GOOD FOR ME TO SPEAK TO:

_____

_____

_____

_____

_____

TO KEEP MENTALLY WELL, I WILL CARRY ON DOING THE THINGS I ENJOY, WHICH ARE:

_____

_____

_____

_____

_____

_____

_____

_____

Conclusion

Adam: Congratulations! You've made it to the end of this book! I hope you've found it helpful, inspiring and, above all, life-changing. Whether you're a young person, or a parent of a younger child with anxiety, worry or OCD and you've taken these steps to create a new story for your thoughts, you'll be in a much better place as a result. And I'd like to add, I admire you from the bottom of my heart. I wish so much that I'd been able to read a book like this when I was younger; if I had, I would have enjoyed a life free from anxiety, worry, and crippling OCD.

When I recovered, I made a promise to pass on the knowledge I'd gained about my illness. This book (plus our companion book for adults) is the result of that promise. OCD has taken me to some very dark places indeed, but it has also been the inspiration for this book and our recovery approach, which we hope will be used right across the world.

As you know now, the root of our strategy to get better lies with three words:

- **Accept**
- **Embrace**
- **Control**

By **accepting** our worries and anxieties for what they are, we no longer need to run away from them. Instead, we **embrace** them, and by hugging them close to us, we learn to **control** them. You have now learned that the secret to controlling our intrusive thoughts is actually to not control them in the conventional sense. And I think this is the most eye-opening secret in our book. If you understand this concept, you have the key to conquering your anxiety, worry, and OCD right at your fingertips.

When I first met Lauren and she told me that, rather than fighting my OCD, panic and anxiety, I'd be better off accepting it, I thought she was joking.

'What a cop out!' I told myself when she'd gone. 'How can I accept something I've been fighting all these years? I need to find a solution to my problem – anything else is just giving in.'

I saw my illness as a 'fight', a 'battle' and a 'struggle' and for all my life I'd responded by putting up my fists and trying to fight back. To be told to lay down my arms and accept the situation as it was seemed ridiculous. There was no way I was going to 'accept' anything about OCD and anxiety.

At that point however, I was so poorly and so in need of help that I had to trust someone. Lauren is one of the leading therapists in anxiety, and I was very fortunate to be able to bring her into my life. If I couldn't trust her, I couldn't trust anyone. She was my last chance. Lauren didn't promise me a miracle cure, but there was a part of me that said, 'Stick with this, and see what happens ...' And I'm so glad that I did because if I'd carried on fighting, battling and struggling I might not be writing these words today.

At one point during the first couple of sessions, Lauren said: 'Adam, everything you thought would be helpful over the last 30 years in trying to fight your mental health issues – has any of it ever worked?'

'I suppose so,' I replied, 'but only for a bit.'

'Okay,' she said, 'then you've been trying to figure this out for more than 30 years and it's made you very ill. So why not try it another way – even if it feels uncomfortable?'

So I thought about it, and just decided to give it a go. As you've been reading, you might have had the same thoughts about this book – but you've stuck with us and made it to the end. Perhaps what you've read has made you feel uncomfortable. Maybe you thought it was strange that we've asked you to accept and embrace your illness for what it is. But, from experience, I know that accepting, embracing and controlling is the only way you will get better.

Acceptance is NOT about giving in. It is about allowing your mind to be how it wants to be, to go where it wants to go, to let in what it wants to let in – thoughts both welcome and unwelcome. It's about saying, 'This is my state of mind, these are the thoughts I am having, this is how I am feeling. I'm accepting my feelings for what they are. I might feel bad, but I accept that.' Until you start 'accepting' it, you are always going to carry the burden of the thoughts and feelings around with you, and over time they will get heavier and heavier.

Think of it like this: If you hold a glass of water in your hand for a short period of time it is quite easy and painless to hold. But if you carry on holding that same glass of water for a much longer period, then it becomes heavier. Even though a glass of water is relatively light, you have continued to hold it for so long that the strain of holding it makes it feel heavier and heavier. It begins to take its toll on your arm muscles. Your physical limits have been stretched and the muscles in your arm simply give up!

So the same applies to your mind trying to cope with your thoughts; if you continue to carry the worries or intrusive thoughts by battling with them, judging them, trying to understand them, or developing a habit to try and make peace with them, then you are continuously carrying them, just like the glass of water. Your mind will only be able to carry them for so long, as I found out when the thoughts just got too heavy and the panic attacks kicked in. Accept your thoughts and state of mind for what they are in that moment, in that hour, day or even that week. Put the glass of water down and go about your day.

Acceptance isn't about fighting, battling or anything else other than having the courage to accept what is. Fight, as we will see, only feeds anxiety. Anxiety loves nothing more than a good battle, because that's where it gains its power. Acceptance is an enemy of anxiety because it diminishes its power. Having the courage to accept your situation is the polar opposite of battling it.

Below is a table of anxiety's likes and dislikes which I've personally found very useful:

WHAT ANXIETY LIKES	WHAT ANXIETY DOESN'T LIKE
• Seeking constant reassurance	• Taking risks with your anxieties
• Performing rituals or compulsions	• Telling your anxiety to 'come on in'
• Running away from your anxiety	• Having the courage to face your fears
• Questioning your state of mind	• Accepting your state of mind
• Fighting or battling your thoughts	• Sitting with your thoughts until they pass
• Feeling uncomfortable about feeling uncomfortable	• Being okay with not feeling okay
• Fearing anxiety	• Doing everyday things despite feeling anxious
• Avoiding everyday things because you feel anxious	• Having compassion for yourself – not judging or blaming
• Trying to 'solve' or figure everything out	• Accepting the uncomfortable feelings and thoughts, knowing they will pass
• Worrying that you will go mad with worry	• Accepting the moment is impermanent

So if you accept your state of mind, and your emotional state, it means you're owning it for what it is. You're not forcing it to do anything; you're simply allowing your anxiety to come and go. I'll be honest; even when I started to understand the concept of **'accept'** there were times it didn't feel right. I reverted to type, put up a fight, and guess what? I felt twice as bad as I did when I was just accepting my state of mind. So eventually I saw it as a 'what will be, will be' moment; a way of letting go of the fight. There was no point fighting, or trying to figure it all out. All that was doing – all it had ever done – was make it worse.

Once I understood this, everything started to become clearer. Acceptance doesn't cure you, but neither does it allow anxiety, worry, and OCD to grow any further. You will still feel anxiety, but as Lauren has demonstrated, this decreases bit by bit over time. This is because you're no longer feeding it by fighting it or reassuring it – you're just accepting what it is, in all its various forms.

A word of warning, though: don't fall into the trap of using the concept of 'acceptance' as a safety behaviour. Don't say to yourself, 'I'm accepting, I'm accepting ...' because that will become a compulsion. True acceptance is NOT telling yourself that it's acceptance. It's about feeling it, just letting it be there, for however long it wants to stay.

I'd say it took me about a month to come to terms with what acceptance is. After that point, I found acceptance coming into my life quite naturally. That was the stage when I knew I was accepting things, but wasn't analysing why and how I was accepting them.

All thoughts, whether good or bad, come from the same place in the brain. I accept the good thoughts – and the nice emotions which are associated with them. By approaching my unwanted and intrusive thoughts in exactly the same way, they started to come and go just as easily as my good thoughts. It felt incredibly liberating. Nothing could harm me, because I didn't care whether it did or it didn't. For the first time in my life, no matter what was being thrown at me, my reaction was simply 'Shove it'. From that point onwards, I started my recovery. Once you accept 'acceptance' you too will begin your journey to recovery and a better life ahead.

Lauren and Adam

We both hope that the journey we've taken you on has been useful, rewarding and life-changing. We know how difficult it is to start on this journey; how challenging it can be to accept and embrace everything we've talked about, and apply it to your own situation. But we also know that to do this successfully can bring untold rewards in terms of a life free from anxiety, worry, OCD, panic attacks and related depression.

By following this approach you get your life back – AND you discover whole new avenues of experience available to you – so it's a double benefit! Taking control of anxiety and freeing yourself from its power is extremely liberating, so be prepared to discover 'a new you' that is ready to open doors, take opportunities and explore new ways of living. Our approach and its principles are not just about survival and recovery, they will help you create a future in the place beyond recovery.

As Adam has said above, if you've followed our book carefully, you will know that at its heart are the concepts of **'ACCEPT'**, **'EMBRACE'** and **'CONTROL'**. We outlined these concepts very carefully and we appreciate that, at first, there is a lot to take in. The good news is, however, that once you have an understanding of Accept-Embrace-Control and are able to implement it into your recovery – and you are able to see the thoughts for what they are – you will be able to use our approach as soon as you notice anxiety creeping in. In time, this will naturally reduce intrusive thoughts and worries.

Now let's recap on some of the main points in this book, so you can refer to them easily as you go through your recovery process and beyond. The 'beyond' bit is particularly important, as there are many lessons contained in these pages that point the way to a life that can be led with more happiness and success … Think of the book as a manual not only for survival and recovery, but also as a handbook for leading a more fulfilled life generally, using our simple, but highly effective approach.

- **ANXIETY** is a response to something we consider to be threatening.
- We all experience anxiety (and worry and fear) at all times in our lives.
- What goes hand-in-hand with anxiety is a feeling that something bad will happen. This feeling has an effect on how our body responds, and in what ways.
- **WORRIES** are the thoughts that you have and ANXIETY describes the emotions and bodily symptoms you feel as a result of those worries.

- **OCD** is an obsessional disorder based in anxiety, in which sufferers attach importance to unwanted thoughts, feelings, images, sensations and urges.

- OCD sufferers employ different strategies (including compulsions, rituals, safety behaviours and reassurance) to reduce anxiety and prevent the feared outcome by trying to get rid of or 'neutralise' the thoughts, feelings, images, sensations and urges.

- The intrusive thought, feeling, image, sensation or urge goes away and you're safe – but only until the next time it pops into your head and causes you distress.

- **PANIC ATTACKS** are part of your emotional and bodily reaction to worry, anxiety or OCD, and are the body's way of protecting itself from things it sees as a 'threat'.

Anxiety and worry occurs for all sorts of reasons and it is common. What makes it a problem is when we give it an importance that has a **significant** effect on our lives. It might prevent us from doing things we previously enjoyed, or it might force us to avoid situations and people. It might also demand that we carry out rituals and behaviours to prevent the feared outcome from happening.

Anxiety, worry, and OCD have various causes, **but they are not your fault**. Anxiety itself is a primal response to threat, better known as 'fight, flight or freeze'. It's a defence mechanism and we all need a little anxiety in our lives to keep us functioning actively. However, anxiety becomes 'dangerous' when we attach importance to it that makes it grow stronger. Attempting to control unhelpful or unwanted thoughts, pushing them aside, inventing safety behaviours to suppress them, or avoiding situations in which they may occur, actually makes problems with anxiety, worry, and OCD much worse.

We call these kinds of responses to thoughts compulsions, or rituals, or safety behaviours. People with OCD and / or anxiety seek comfort in compulsions and safety behaviours because they see them as ways around their worries. They can be both physical and mental. We call them **'safety behaviours'** because they are actions that anxiety sufferers carry out to feel safe from the feared outcome. This might bring relief at first, but the anxiety will not go away altogether, and will need more rituals, compulsions, safety behaviours, avoidance and reassurance to keep warding off the anxiety. These techniques only reinforce the strength of the 'Worst-Case Scenario' meaning, bringing increasing anxiety and disturbance to everyday life.

As we've mentioned, our approach has, at its core, three principal concepts: Accept, Embrace and Control.

- We **accept** that we all have worries and fears, and experience anxiety, and we understand that is our current state of mind. We do not question or fight our state of mind; instead, *we allow it to be what it is*.

- We face our worries and fears, **embrace** them, move towards them and let them in. We do not 'run away' by distracting ourselves, avoiding them or doing other things to keep ourselves and others safe.

- We eventually learn how to **control** our mental health and see it for what it is without judging it – a collection of thoughts and feelings; no more, no less. 'Control' means accepting that it's okay not to be in control of your thoughts and the sensations and emotions attached to them.

Once you have begun your journey to recovery, you may start asking yourself ... is that it? Is that all there is to this – Accept, Embrace, Control? Well, yes, that's it! There's no point questioning how simple this is. Instead, accept and embrace it by facing your fears and have the courage to see it through.

When faced with worry and anxiety, your mind tries to persuade you to fight, run away or freeze. So do the opposite – accept and embrace it. Doing this is the only way to control it and make a full recovery. Have courage and take the journey – you will never look back.

We sincerely hope you've enjoyed the journey we've shared with you in this book and the approach contained within it. You now have the tools and the inspiration you need to embark on your own journey out of the grip of anxiety, OCD and panic attacks. We hope that your journey is a fruitful one, and that it leads to a life of peace, contentment and fulfilment. Recovery can be inevitable, we promise.

You'll find more information at: **www.trigger-press.com**

Please sign up to our charity, The Shaw Mind Foundation, (**www.shawmindfoundation.org**) and keep in touch with us, we'd love to hear from you.

*"We aim to bring to an end the suffering and despair caused
by mental health issues. Our goal is to make help and support
available for every single person in society, from all walks of life.
We will never stop offering hope. These are our promises.'*

Trigger Press and The Shaw Mind Foundation

Join us and follow us...

@trigger_press
@Shaw_Mind

Search **The Shaw Mind Foundation** on Facebook
Search **Trigger Press** on Facebook

Notes

1   **Shafran, R., Thordarson, D. S., & Rachman, S.** (1996). 'Thought-action fusion in obsessive compulsive disorder'. *Journal of Anxiety Disorders*, 10(5), 379–91.

2   **Salkovskis, P. M., Wroe, A. L., Gledhill, A., Morrison, N., Forrester, E., Richards, C., & Thorpe, S.** (2000). 'Responsibility attitudes and interpretations are characteristic of obsessive compulsive disorder'. *Behaviour Research and Therapy*, 38(4), 347–72.

3   Adapted from **Uher, R., Heyman, I., Mortimer, C., Frampton, I. & Goodman, R.** (2007) 'Screening young people for obsessive compulsive disorder'. *British Journal of Psychiatry*, 191, 353–4. Also available online at www.ocdyouth.iop.kcl.ac.uk/downloads/socs.pdf.

4   **Clark, D. M.** (1986). 'A cognitive approach to panic'. *Behaviour Research and Therapy*, 24(4), 461–70.

Bibliography

American Psychiatric Association. (2013). 'Diagnostic and Statistical Manual of Mental Disorders' (5th ed.). Washington, DC: American Psychiatric Association.

Clark, D. M. (1989) 'Anxiety states: Panic and generalized anxiety'. In Hawton, K., Salkovskis, P. M., Kirk, J. & Clark, D. M. (eds). *Cognitive Behaviour Therapy for Psychiatric Problems: A Practical Guide*. New York, NY, US: Oxford University Press, pp. 52–96.

Gilbert, P. (2010). *The Compassionate Mind: A New Approach to Life's Challenge*. Oakland, CA: New Harbinger Publications.

Salkovskis, P. M. (1985). 'Obsessive-compulsive problems: A cognitive behavioural analysis'. *Behaviour Research and Therapy*, 11, 271–7.

Salkovskis, P. M. (1999). 'Understanding and treating obsessive-compulsive disorder'. *Behaviour Research and Therapy*, 37, S29–S52.

Salkovskis, P. M., Wroe, A. L., Gledhill, A., Morrison, N., Forrester, E., Richards, C., & Thorpe, S. (2000). 'Responsibility attitudes and interpretations are characteristic of obsessive compulsive disorder'. *Behaviour Research and Therapy*, 38(4), 347–72.

Shafran, R., Thordarson, D. S. & Rachman, S. (1996). 'Thought-action fusion in obsessive compulsive disorder'. *Journal of Anxiety Disorders*, 10(5), 379–91.

Stallard, P. (2008). *Anxiety: Cognitive Behaviour Therapy with Children and Young People*. Hove: Routledge.

Stallard, P. (2009). 'Cognitive behaviour therapy with children and young people'. In Beinart, H. & Kennedy, D. (eds), *Clinical Psychology in Practice*. Chichester: BPS Blackwell, pp. 117–26.

Uher, R., Heyman, I., Mortimer, C., Frampton, I. & Goodman, R. (2007) 'Screening young people for obsessive compulsive disorder'. *British Journal of Psychiatry,* 191, 353–4. Also available online at www.ocdyouth.iop.kcl.ac.uk/downloads/socs.pdf.

Index

TRIGGERPRESS

Giving mental health a voice

www.trigger-press.com

Trigger Press is a publishing house devoted to opening conversations about mental health. We tell the stories of people who have suffered from mental illnesses and recovered, so that others may learn from them.

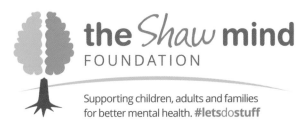

the *Shaw* mind
FOUNDATION

Supporting children, adults and families
for better mental health. **#letsdostuff**

Sign up to our charity, The Shaw Mind Foundation

www.shawmindfoundation.org

and keep in touch with us; we would love to hear from you.

We aim to bring to an end the suffering and despair caused
by mental health issues. Our goal is to make help and support
available for every single person in society, from all walks of life.
We will never stop offering hope. These are our promises.

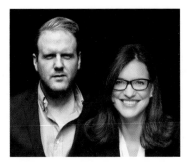

Adam Shaw is a worldwide mental health advocate and philanthropist. Now in recovery from mental health issues, he is committed to helping others suffering from debilitating mental health issues through the global charity he co-founded, The Shaw Mind Foundation. www.shawmindfoundation.org

Lauren Callaghan (CPsychol, PGDipClinPsych, PgCert, MA (hons), LLB (hons), BA), born and educated in New Zealand, is an innovative industry-leading psychologist based in London, United Kingdom. Lauren has worked with children and young people, and their families, in a number of clinical settings providing evidence based treatments for a range of illnesses, including anxiety and obsessional problems. She was a psychologist at the specialist national treatment centres for severe obsessional problems in the UK and is renowned as an expert in the field of mental health, recognised for diagnosing and successfully treating OCD and anxiety related illnesses in particular. In addition to appearing as a treating clinician in the critically acclaimed and BAFTA award-winning documentary *Bedlam*, Lauren is a frequent guest speaker on mental health conditions in the media and at academic conferences. Lauren also acts as a guest lecturer and honorary researcher at the Institute of Psychiatry Kings College, UCL.

Additional copies of the tables from this book can be downloaded from the Trigger Press website.

Please visit the link below:

www.trigger-press.com/resources